The Life and Death of Lumpy Parker

A Story of Sarcoma Survival

Christi Parker

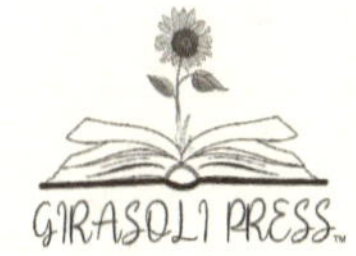
GIRASOLI PRESS

To my dearest Blaine, whose unwavering faith held us both up when I thought we might drown. You will forever be my very favorite person.

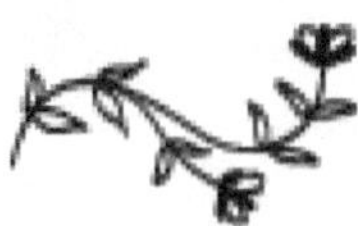

To our amazing girls, Kaia, Kaci, and Kamryn. You stepped into adulthood long before I hoped with grace and maturity. Never forget how strong you are.

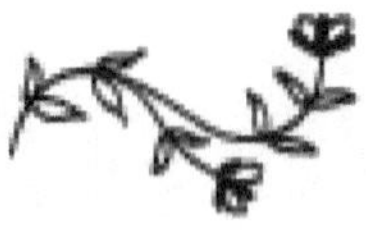

To my friends who were family who fought this fight first, Bucky, Kathy, Lori, Preston, and Stephanie. You taught me what true bravery and strength look like. I miss you.

"Cancer is stupid. And inconvenient. Avoid it."
—Stephanie Fredrick

Chapter 1

I paused my early-morning rush to gaze at the snowflakes drifting peacefully to the ground as if they weren't going to band together to cause complete chaos.

"That's weird. I have this little lump on my arm."

I turned to see my husband, Blaine, walk in rubbing his arm.

"Let me see." I moved his arm around, but didn't notice anything unusual.

"Here," he said, placing my finger on his upper arm. Sure enough, there was something under the skin. It was tiny, about the size of a small pea. You couldn't see it, but you could feel it.

"Does it hurt?"

"No, not at all."

"Yeah, that's weird," I said as I moved past him to get my shoes, not having any idea the snow was going to be the least of my worries.

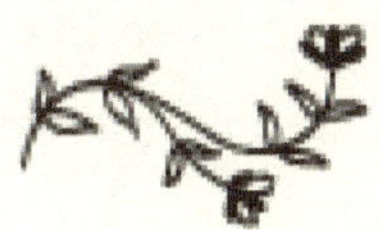

It was my favorite time of the year, the week between Christmas and New Year's. Kaia, our oldest daughter, was a freshman in college. We were a homeschooling family, and I spent almost every day with our girls. Under the best of situations, having our first child move away would be hard, but it was 2020, and Kaia was on the school's gymnastics team. The COVID restrictions placed on college athletes meant we were not allowed to see her.

Thankfully, the coach decided families could visit for Christmas as long as we kept the girls isolated. I had found the cutest little cabin, and we had spent four perfect days together as a family. Now the rest of us were back home, but competition season started in a week, and we would be able to see Kaia many times through the spring. It would have to be from a distance, but that was better than nothing.

Life was good. I was happy. Everything was just as it should be.

Except it wasn't.

Over the next couple weeks, the tiny lump grew. Soon it was noticeable just by looking at Blaine's arm. I Googled "lump on arm" and saw the word *sarcoma*, possibly for the first time. Fear jolted through me, but then I read on to learn sarcomas are extremely rare. I am a worrier by nature, but according to the website, it seemed the chances of my young, healthy husband having a sarcoma were almost impossible.

The lump continued to grow.

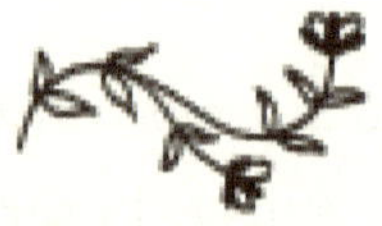

I was making dinner one evening when Blaine walked in from work. He leaned down to give me a kiss and then dropped a bomb: "I think I need to see a doctor about my arm."

My heart skipped a beat. Blaine and I had been married for twenty-three years, and he had never once thought he should see a doctor. Whereas I tend to think everything is serious, Blaine thinks nothing is.

"I think you should go with me."

"Okay," I replied calmly, like he hadn't just completely knocked the wind out of me. Wanting to see a doctor *and* wanting me to go with him must mean he was worried. Somehow my sarcoma fear no longer seemed so impossible. I made the appointment and started researching. The statistics for sarcomas are not good.

We had actually been down this road before. The year we were married, Blaine's mother found a lump on her neck. She went to the doctor, who told her it was just a swollen lymph node. She took antibiotics, but it kept growing. She returned again and again, somehow knowing it was more serious, but was repeatedly assured it was nothing to worry about. Finally, the doctor agreed to biopsy the lump. He discovered it was cancer and said she only had about five years to live. He was wrong. She died three months later.

With Blaine's family history and the sarcoma statistics swirling in my head, we went in for his appointment two days later. We sat in the waiting room, the knot in my stomach growing larger, until the nurse called his name and led us to the exam room.

"What brings you in today, Mr. Parker?"

"This." He pointed to the now quite visible lump on his arm.

"Oh! You have a lipoma!"

I was skeptical of her ability to diagnose medical conditions by glancing at them but started to feel just a little bit better. Maybe I was wrong after all.

The doctor walked in and looked at it. "Oh! You have a lipoma!"

He sounded completely confident and the knot in my stomach relaxed. "How exactly do you know it's a lipoma and not a sarcoma?" I asked.

He listed several logical reasons. He mentioned it being squishy and mobile and tried to assure us that worrisome lumps weren't squishy or mobile. Everything he said made sense, but we knew the doctors seeing Blaine's mom had made sense as well. We talked about her and about how the doctors were confident she didn't have anything concerning.

"If the lump were on Blaine's neck, then I would be more worried, but based on how squishy it is and the location, I'm sure it's nothing at all to worry about. If you would like, I will order an ultrasound so we can be doubly sure, but those are fairly expensive, and I already know what it will show."

We trusted the doctor. There was no point in spending money just to confirm what he had already told us. We left his office, and I felt the weight of the world had completely lifted from my shoulders. I felt so silly for worrying and jumped right back into life, not thinking about Blaine's arm at all.

The lump continued to grow, and being the original and creative people we are, we started calling it Lumpy.

A couple weeks passed, and the day came for Blaine's annual physical. By now, Lumpy was considerably bigger, but the doctor continued to remain confident it was just a lipoma. He did offer to ultrasound it again. He even offered to just have it cut off because it was getting pretty ugly, but he assured Blaine it was absolutely nothing to worry about.[1] Blaine declined.

Life went on, and it was complicated enough without overthinking Blaine's arm. We watched Kaia fall at a competition on TV. She seriously injured her elbow and had to have surgery to repair it. Kaci, our middle daughter, was a senior in high school. She had been training most of her life to become a professional ballet dancer and had already secured a prestigious internship with her dream company, but she had hurt her hip, and we weren't sure what that meant for her future. Kamryn, our youngest, was a busy eighth grader, leading an active social life. I was juggling teaching two grades, dealing with the injuries, and trying desperately to get enough actual paying work done to help with the expenses. Life was stressful.

Lumpy continued to grow. Now it was quite large. Finally, Blaine decided just to go ahead and have it removed, and I made an appointment with a general surgeon. We were not happy to be spending the money but were looking forward to its being gone. I picked Blaine up at his office. He told the owners of the company he would be back in a couple of hours. We talked about having lunch before he went back to work. Both of us completely expected they would numb him up and slice off the lump and we would be on our way.

We were wrong.

Chapter 2

The physician's assistant came into the room to cut off Lumpy. She took one look at it and froze. "That's not a lipoma."

"What do you mean? My doctor was sure it was just a lipoma."

"It's not. Look how red it is. This is a hemangioma. It's filled with blood vessels, and we can't cut it off without knowing exactly where they are. The doctor needs to look at this." She left the room and in a surprisingly short amount of time returned with the doctor.

He walked over and pushed all around Lumpy. "Does it hurt?"

"No, not a bit."

"Well, it's definitely not a lipoma. If we cut into that here, you will bleed out on the table and we won't be able to stop it. We need an ultrasound to show us exactly where the blood vessels are, and we're going to have to do the surgery at the hospital."

With that one sentence, what we thought was a moderately expensive issue became a major problem. I fought hard to keep from panicking as I thought of all the money we needed. Kaia had just had surgery. Now Blaine needed one, and I suspected Kaci was going to as well. Our insurance didn't pay a dime until we reached our very large deductible. Somehow, even though our children have always been very active in sports, our family has been blessed with good health, and we have never had to deal with large medical expenses. It seemed our luck had run out. Where would we get the money to pay for all of this? I choked down my worry and shot Blaine what I hoped was a reassuring smile.

It turned out money wasn't going to be the only problem with getting rid of Lumpy. COVID was making everything more complicated. We lived in an area that remained reasonably normal during the pandemic, but it did slow things down. While getting an appointment for a medical test normally would take just a couple of days, it took a couple of weeks to get in for the ultrasound.

Finally, the morning of Blaine's appointment arrived, and we walked up to the desk to check in. The receptionist took all of his information and said, "That will be $500."

I swallowed hard. I knew it was going to be expensive, but it hadn't occurred to me they would expect payment upfront. "We'd like to wait and pay that after it goes through our insurance," Blaine told her.

She tilted her head and looked up at us through squinting eyes. "That's not how we normally do things."

"Okay," I flashed my sweetest smile. "But that's how we're going to do it today."

She sighed and punched a few buttons on her keyboard. "Fine. Sit over there. They'll let you know when they're ready."[2]

A nurse called Blaine's name a few minutes later and took him back for the procedure. It was quick and painless, and we walked out of the building thirty minutes after we walked in, assuming Lumpy would be cut off later that week.

Instead, a few days later, the physician's assistant called. "I'm sorry Mrs. Parker, but the results of the ultrasound were inconclusive. We need an MRI to really be able to see where the blood vessels are."

I could feel my blood pressure rising. Another delay. More money. This was getting completely out of hand considering it was just some excess tissue. "Are you absolutely sure you can't just go ahead and cut it off?"

"I'm afraid we can't. We have to know exactly what we're cutting into. Blaine could bleed to death if we cut the wrong place."

I sank into a chair and racked my brain, trying to think of an effective argument, but, of course, got nothing. I would never consider risking his life just to save some money. "Okay," I sighed. "Go ahead and schedule it."

Getting on the MRI calendar took a few more weeks, but finally it was done, and we just needed to wait for the results. While we were getting tests done on Lumpy, Kaci's hip was getting worse. She had an MRI of her own, and the results were much worse than we had feared. The cartilage lining her joint was torn almost all the way around. None of the surgeons near us had seen anything like it, so I expanded the search to bigger cities. I finally found one three hours away who specialized in dance injuries and had fixed hips like Kaci's many times. It seemed crazy that we would have to drive that far for medical care, but it was the only option. We made plans for surgery in June. We wanted to let her get through her high school graduation and eighteenth birthday on two feet.

By this time, it was mid-May and time to bring Kaia home for the summer! She had only been gone for nine months, but it felt like years. Blaine and I decided to leave a day early and attend a festival near Kaia's college town. We hadn't been anywhere overnight without the girls in thirteen years, and it seemed like the perfect opportunity. I couldn't keep the grin off my face as I rambled on and on about how much I was looking forward to our time together and to the rest of the summer.

We had only been on the road for an hour when my phone rang. I sucked in my breath when I recognized Kaci's surgeon's number. I showed Blaine the phone. "This can't be good," I grumbled as I pushed the button to answer.

I wasn't wrong. The surgeon's assistant got right to the point. "I'm afraid we have a problem. The physical therapist called this morning. She's worried Kaci's cartilage is tearing further. Dr. Smith says we need to do the surgery within the next week, or she is at risk for doing permanent damage." My heart sank. So much for Kaci's easy graduation celebration.

So much also for the long drive just enjoying the scenery and the uninterrupted conversations with my husband I had been looking forward to.

Instead, I spent the next five hours on the phone going back and forth with all the people involved in performing major orthopedic surgery. We had been expecting a relatively simple procedure and recovery period at a conveniently scheduled time. Instead, our seventeen-year-old daughter was going to have major hip surgery involving at least one overnight hospital stay, a big, ugly brace, and a prolonged, complicated rehabilitation period.

I finished with the last of the details and we checked into our bed and breakfast. Blaine and I stuffed our anxiety about Kaci and enjoyed our time at the festival. At some point during the evening, he grabbed my hand and smiled. "We really should make a point to get away together more often."

The next morning, we finished making our way to Kaia. I hadn't seen her since her surgery eight weeks earlier, and Blaine hadn't seen her since Christmas. We had a great time catching up, and I was so excited for all of us to be back together. Once we got past Kaci's surgery, I was sure the summer was going to be awesome!

Chapter 3

Two days later, I was driving home with Kaci when I remembered I had received an email saying Blaine's MRI results were in. I glanced over and saw she was looking at her phone. "Oh, hey, can you log into Dad's health account and see what his MRI showed?" We had been assured so many times by so many doctors that Lumpy was nothing to worry about, it didn't even cross my mind the report could contain bad news.

I pulled off the highway onto the exit nearest our house as she opened the results. "Undifferentiated pleomorphic sarcoma versus myxoid liposarcoma. Referral to orthopedic oncologist is recommended."

Fear like a dark, heavy blanket wrapped around me. I could feel my heart beating, my lungs breathing, every centimeter of my skin. My mind raced with a million thoughts and was absolutely blank at the same time.

"What's a sarcoma?" she asked.

I couldn't answer her. I sat in stunned silence, unable to force out the words. Finally, my brain and mouth reconnected. "I am pretty sure that's cancer."

She didn't move. She didn't make a sound. The *C* word hung in the air like a physical presence. "I'm sure it's fine," I gushed. "It's just on his arm. They'll just cut the lump off, and it will all be fine." I paused and tried to grasp the fact that I had just let my child discover her father had cancer. "Don't tell your sisters yet."

Now I had let my child discover her dad had cancer *and* made her keep a secret from her sisters. Mother of the Year right here.

As we pulled into our garage, my phone rang. Kaci fled into the house while I picked it up and gave a shaky "Hello?"

"Hey!" my friend, Carolyn, said. "How's your day going?"

Silence.

Finally, I forced myself to speak. "I think Blaine has cancer." The word *cancer* felt like gravel in my mouth. I thought I might actually gag just saying it out loud. Carolyn was silent while I babbled on. "I let Kaci read the report . . . I thought it was nothing . . . I'm sure it's fine . . . How could I let her be the one to read it? . . . They're probably wrong . . . I'm sure they'll just cut it off . . . How do we tell the girls? . . . I'm sure it's fine." I just kept talking, like somehow I could chase away the monster we were facing if I threw enough words at it.

I was still rambling a few minutes later when my phone beeped, and I looked down to see the physician's assistant was calling. Without a word to Carolyn, I switched lines. I didn't even say hello. "I thought I might be hearing from you."

"I take it you've seen the report?"

"Yes. What in the world? Everyone said it was fine."

"We had our suspicions but were hoping we were wrong. We need to get this taken care of quickly, but no one in Springfield will touch a sarcoma. You're going to have to go to St. Louis."

A dark shadow fell over me as her words sank in. Springfield, Missouri isn't a large city, but it has well-respected medical facilities. People only sought treatment out of town for extremely serious conditions. We were already going out of town for Kaci's hip. My mind couldn't grasp that we were now going to have to go away for Blaine's treatment as well—and to the opposite side of the state from where Kaci was going to be. Two days ago our lives had been totally fine; now they seemed to be completely falling apart. I fought for breath as the waves of bad news hit me all at once.

The PA asked if I wanted her to call Blaine or if I wanted to tell him myself. I had trouble deciding, but eventually asked her to call him in case he had questions I wouldn't be able to answer. I hung up the phone and numbly went to prepare dinner, trying unsuccessfully to keep my mind away from the image of Blaine hearing the news and the conversation we were sure to have when he got home.

He walked into the house a little while later and bent down to kiss me. "How was your day?" he asked the same way he always did.

I stared at him. He must not know our world had just been shattered. I stood still a few more moments, trying to decide what to say and then finally asked, "Did the PA call you?"

"Yes."

"And?"

"And what?"

"How are you feeling? What are you thinking?"

"I'm not happy, but it will be fine. It's on my arm. They'll just take it off."

And with those words, I felt better again. Blaine has always been very practical. In his mind, God is in control and nothing is ever an actual problem. You do what you need to and just keep going. My mind tends to jump to the worst possible scenario, to play out horrible outcomes and situations, but Blaine can almost always bring me back down. Even though he was the one who was actually going to have to endure whatever treatment was needed, he was the one assuring me that everything would work out. I told him about Kaci reading the MRI report and that we needed to tell Kaia and Kamryn quickly so she didn't have to keep the secret.

As soon as all three girls were home, we called them into the living room and asked them to sit down. "Oooohhhh!" Kaia said. "The last time you called a meeting in the living room, you announced we were going to Disneyland!"

I took a deep breath and fought to control my voice. "We're not going to Disneyland."

The air suddenly felt heavier. Kaia and Kamryn looked at us expectantly. Kaci focused on the floor, refusing to look up. Blaine and I looked at each other, realizing we should have planned this better.

He took the plunge. "You know how the doctors were sure Lumpy was not a problem?" Both girls nodded their heads slowly. "It turns out they were probably wrong." He paused. Somehow the air felt even heavier. He took a deep breath. "They think it is probably cancer."

Kaia and Kamryn sat perfectly still, keeping their eyes glued on their father. Kaci finally looked up to see their reaction. They didn't say a word. It seemed that no one was even breathing.

"I know that sounds scary, but everything will be fine. We will have to go to a hospital in St. Louis, but they'll just cut it off, and we'll go on with our lives."

"But . . . what about Grandma?" Kamryn whispered softly.

"This isn't like that," I rushed to assure her. "It's just on his arm. They'll just take it off."

They asked a few more questions, and we continued to confirm that everything was going to be fine. We were being completely honest with them, but it turned out we had an awful lot to learn about sarcomas.

Chapter 4

Even though my head told me Blaine would most likely be fine, my heart wasn't convinced. The fear that had latched on the moment I heard the word *sarcoma* refused to leave. Fear was quickly joined by sadness. I didn't want to walk the road we were facing. I wanted my life back. I had no idea what our next week would look like, not to mention the next ten years. I was a planner who had no way to plan. I ached to wake up and discover all of it had been just a bad dream.

The PA told me on the phone that she would call Trinity Hospital in St. Louis and make a referral immediately. She said we would hear from them soon. I fully expected a call the next morning. It didn't come. I waited all day, but no call from Trinity. My husband had cancer that had been growing inside him for who knows how long because the doctors had misdiagnosed it, and now *another* full day had gone by with no one stepping up to take care of it.

Blaine is a very private person. He has always been uncomfortable with people outside our immediate family knowing what was happening with him. When we told the girls he had cancer, he immediately asked them not to tell anyone. Later I convinced him they really needed to be able to talk about their feelings with someone, so he agreed they could each tell one person. My friend who happened to call immediately after Kaci read the report knew, and I did tell a few other friends who had unique experiences with cancer, but for the most part, our little family just went about our business like everything was fine. Almost no one had any idea what we were facing. There were times, even after we understood the seriousness of our reality, that we had long conversations with close friends and never once even hinted there was anything wrong with our lives. It makes me wonder, "How many other people I encounter every day are also dealing with crises I have no idea about?"

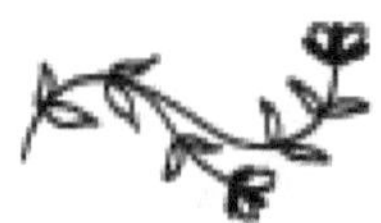

Another day went by with no call from Trinity. I carried my phone around, obsessively checking to make sure I hadn't missed a call. Then *another* day went by. Three full days had passed from the time we learned the doctors had made a major mistake with Blaine's care, and no one was doing anything to take care of it. Surely, there must have been a mistake with the referral; so, I called the surgeon's office to ask them to check on it. My heart stopped beating when the scheduler explained how referrals worked.

"They have thirty days to contact you to schedule a consultation."

I thought I had misunderstood her, but, no, I had heard correctly. Even though the medical establishment had let this thing grow inside Blaine's body for several months, assuring us it was fine while it just continued to get bigger and bigger, they now had *another* full month before they even had to call to schedule an appointment to *talk* about taking care of it. Based on how long it took just to get the MRI and ultrasound scheduled, I knew it would likely take a very long time to get an appointment with an actual surgeon, and they had twenty-seven more days to even contact us.

I started crying on the phone. I am *not* a crier, and I certainly *never* cry in front of other people. I just don't. I convinced myself years ago that crying does nothing helpful and decided I just wouldn't do it. I had not cried about Blaine's having cancer at all up to this point, but I lost it on the phone.

Trinity called to schedule the appointment the next day.

After I learned that Trinity Hospital had so long to respond to the referral, I decided to check on MD Anderson in Houston, Texas. We had always heard amazing things about this hospital, and I had helped take a friend there a few years earlier. I had been amazed at their campus, their resources, and the professionalism of every single staff person I came into contact with. I still did not totally understand that Blaine was indeed facing a serious cancer but decided just to check out their website and see how difficult it might be to get him seen there.

It was shockingly easy. There was literally a button at the top of the website that said, "Request an Appointment." I clicked on it, filled out a tiny bit of basic information, and sent it in. Within hours, Blaine received a call from someone at MD Anderson requesting his medical records and insurance information. Relief and terror flooded my body simultaneously. We were finally getting started.

Chapter 5

The next morning, Kaci and I loaded up the car and drove to Kansas City for her surgery. We met with Dr. Smith, and he went over in detail exactly what he would be doing and what we should expect with her recovery. It was going to be a pretty intense surgery that would take several hours.

We left the surgeon's office feeling optimistic that she would soon have less pain but also fairly depressed. Kaci was in her senior year of high school. She was only seventeen years old. It seemed so bizarre that she was about to have "old lady surgery" (her words). It was also bizarre that this was not the most serious health issue we were facing. I was feeling completely overwhelmed with all of it but did my best to focus on Kaci, and we tried to enjoy her last evening of being able to walk freely. We explored stores we don't have in Springfield and bought a few things for her upcoming graduation party. She ran out of steam early, so we grabbed some dinner and went to bed, ready to get tomorrow over with.

We drove to the hospital early the next morning, and they prepped her for surgery. Thanks to the hospital's COVID rules, the second they took her back to the operating room, they booted me right out of the hospital. They said I was "welcome to wait in the parking lot." Thankfully, our hotel was nearby, so I went back to wait for them to call to tell me she was awake and I could come back. I spent the next several hours praying for my child's surgery and researching cancer hospitals for my husband.

It was nice to have some time to sit and research. By this point, I had learned more about sarcomas, and what I had learned was not good. I hadn't understood why the life expectancy for people with sarcomas was so poor, but I learned that some are extremely aggressive and spread quickly to the patient's lungs and then getting rid of them is very difficult. I had also learned that the methods for treating sarcomas vary widely and it is critically important that patients are seen at a high-volume sarcoma center. Trinity Hospital and MD Anderson were both on the list as being high-volume centers, but MD Anderson was generally recognized as the best. Trinity was three hours from our house. MDA was eleven. Was it worth seeking treatment eleven hours from home? Was there somewhere else that would be better? Were the doctors wrong, and he really didn't have a sarcoma? Were they right, and it had already spread? Did he need chemotherapy? Would they amputate his arm? Was he going to die?

I prayed for wisdom and read everything I could find. I was overwhelmed with the fact that the decisions we made about his care could literally determine whether he lived or died, and there was so much we did not know. I was trying desperately to learn as much as I could, but my brain seemed so sluggish. I had always prided myself on my ability to sort through information and make quick decisions, but now I felt like I was moving in slow motion, that my brain was filled with sludge, and I simply could not think clearly. There had never been a time in my life when it was more important that I make a good decision, so I just kept pushing on.

Eventually the surgeon called and said the surgery had gone well. Kaci would be in recovery for the next few hours, and the nurse would call me when she was in her room and I could go back to the hospital. I called Blaine to let him know the surgery was over and went back to my research. When the nurse called a few hours later, I shifted my mental gears back to Kaci and drove to the hospital. I was so thankful that part of the ordeal was over!

My heart ached when I walked into Kaci's room. She was clearly in tremendous pain, and while I knew she was glad I was there, there was absolutely nothing I could do to help her. She had an IV tube in her arm as well as ice machine tubes going to her hip. There was a big brace around her pelvis and down her leg. Both feet were strapped in boots with a large, hard foam cylinder between them.

I felt a sense of whiplash, this weird shifting in my brain. I had spent the last few hours obsessing over how best to care for my husband, and now I needed to switch and take care of my daughter's serious issues. I didn't know it then, of course, but this jarring of my mental focus from one crisis to another would be repeated over and over and over in the coming months. I would end up feeling like my brain was bruised.

Although the plan had been for Kaci to spend at least one night in the hospital, the forecast for the next day called for torrential rain, so it was decided we should drive home that night. I was pretty nervous taking her home by myself, but we made it just fine, and I was so happy to pull into the garage and be back with the rest of the family!

Chapter 6

Although Kaci's hip pain was completely gone within a couple of days, she still faced six weeks of intense movement restrictions and months of rehab. We had left the hospital with a CPM (continuous passive motion) machine. We had to strap her leg onto the machine, and it gently moved her hip and knee back and forth. She needed to do this for six hours every day. If she wasn't using the CPM, but was sitting or lying down, then her feet always had to be strapped into the immobilization boots. She had anti-inflammatory pills, antibiotic pills, and anti-clotting pills to take multiple times a day. She had a machine that circulated cold water through a pad that was placed on her hip. This had to be refilled every few hours. She had to wear compression socks any time she wasn't in the shower, and getting these on and off her without moving her hip provided me with a full body workout. Of course, she couldn't put any weight on her leg, so she couldn't carry anything and, thus, had to be completely waited on constantly. For the most part, she handled all of this extremely well, but she was still a lot of work!

While my focus had shifted momentarily to caring for Kaci, Trinity Hospital had scheduled Blaine's surgery consultation much quicker than I had expected. In fact, it was the next week. I was so thankful they were now moving quickly, but that meant I was going to have to leave Kaci. Kaia and Kamryn jumped right in to do everything they could to help, and I knew they were very capable, but I was still nervous. So many things could go wrong!

Thankfully, one of our friends is a nurse. She lives close by, and I knew she would be more than happy to help with Kaci if she needed anything. Unfortunately, that meant I would have to explain to her why Blaine and I would be gone. I sent her a text. I simply could not say the words out loud. She immediately responded back that she was sorry about the situation, and, of course, she would be on call to help in any way she could with Kaci. Then, within minutes, she sent us $500.

I froze and stared at the screen showing the money transfer. Somehow it hadn't yet occurred to me that we were truly in a situation in which we needed people to give us money. Other people had those kinds of problems, not us!

I was so touched by this. Our friend saw a need and immediately did what she could to help. I wanted to be this type of giver. I just didn't want to be in a situation in which I was the receiver. I sat there for a few moments, feeling nauseous as I pictured her thinking we needed that kind of money. I quickly wrote back, thanking her for the gift, but telling her we were fine. Then I sent the money back.[3]

Around this time, as I was learning more and more about sarcomas, I felt the overwhelming need to know people were praying for Blaine. People couldn't pray if they didn't know. Blaine still wanted to keep his personal business as private as possible but agreed we needed prayer, so we started telling a few more people, including his closest friends and a few members of his family. I sent texts. I can't imagine how they felt reading someone they loved had cancer. There are some things I did during this time I'm proud of. This is not one of them. I just couldn't imagine saying the words to the people who loved him the most. I mentioned earlier that I am not a crier, but by this point, I was crying pretty easily, and I just knew I would cry while I was talking to them. I couldn't stand that idea. Even though I regret breaking the news through a text, I'm not sure I would do it differently now. Sometimes during a journey like this, you just have to do what you need to do to take care of yourself. For me, I needed to just send texts.

A few days after Kaci's surgery, Blaine and I left to meet with the surgeon in St. Louis. The three-hour drive was uneventful, but as Blaine pulled into the parking lot of the hospital, my mouth fell open, and I leaned over to stare up at the towering, forbidding buildings. I took a slow, deep breath and tried to settle my racing heart as Blaine parked the car and we climbed out. We grabbed each other's hands and walked into another world.

When the Trinity scheduler called, she had informed us Blaine was going to be meeting with the head of surgical oncology. We were so thankful he would be in the best hands! We made our way through the COVID screeners at the door and stopped at the information desk for directions. The inside of the hospital, while bright and sleek looking, was just as imposing as the outside, and I was thankful for the guidance.

We stepped off the elevator and then froze as we read the sign on the wall: "Welcome to the Gastrointestinal Department." I clenched Blaine's hand as my heart began to race with anger. They had set us up with the wrong surgeon! Blaine leaned down and whispered into my ear, "Let's just see what they have to say."

All of the staff acted like it was perfectly normal for a patient with a sarcoma on his arm to be in a GI office. Finally, the surgeon came in and started poking around on Lumpy. "Does it hurt?"

"No, not at all," Blaine replied. We would learn that lots of sarcomas are very painful. We were so thankful Blaine's never hurt him.

"Well, it definitely looks like a sarcoma. We will take it off and then do a biopsy to find out exactly what it is. What the biopsy shows will determine if you need any further treatment."

This is exactly what we were hoping to hear. We just wanted it off. What we didn't want to hear came next: "You'll spend the night in the hospital after the surgery, and then you'll go home with a drain for a few weeks. You'll need to come back here to have the drain removed." Now, on top of the operation, we were looking at hotel rooms, multiple trips, time away from the girls, and a nasty drain. All of this seemed like such a big deal, but we obviously didn't have a choice. They had an opening in the surgery schedule in two weeks, which we gratefully accepted, and then we hurried back home to our girls.

Chapter 7

That weekend was Kaci's much-anticipated high school graduation party. This was complicated by the fact that some of the guests knew about Lumpy, but most did not. We didn't want to take a chance on the focus being taken off Kaci, so we asked those who knew not to mention it. It was amazing to me that the news didn't get out. One family member actually stayed with us for three days, and we kept the secret safe.[4] Kaci's graduation (and eighteenth birthday) weekend went off perfectly. It was a time of relaxation and celebration for all of us. We all needed the time to focus on something besides cancer.

Soon though, it was time to get back to our reality. The day of Blaine's scheduled surgery was getting closer. I continued to read everything I could find on sarcomas, and I started to feel more and more uncomfortable with the plan. Getting Lumpy taken off was exactly what we thought we wanted. If it was indeed cancer, it seemed wise to remove it as quickly as possible. I didn't understand why I felt so ... unsettled, but I did. I just couldn't shake it. Finally, I called Blaine at work and asked if he was positive he hadn't missed a message from MD Anderson. He assured me he hadn't and asked why.

"I can't really explain it. I just keep feeling we're doing the wrong thing, that maybe we shouldn't be getting this taken care of at Trinity."

There was no logical reason for this feeling. Trinity is a very well-respected hospital. It is listed as a high-volume sarcoma center, and while not necessarily a sarcoma specialist, Blaine's doctor was obviously a very experienced surgeon. Plus, we had not heard anything from MD Anderson in a couple of weeks. The surgery was scheduled. We needed to move forward.

I was shocked an hour later when Blaine called. A scheduler from MD Anderson had just called him. Sometime during their initial conversations weeks earlier, Blaine had mentioned he just wasn't sure what to do. She had taken that to mean he wasn't sure he wanted a referral to their hospital, so she hadn't forwarded his information on to the surgeon. She was calling now to see if he wanted her to send it. By this point, Blaine *really* wasn't sure what to do, so he asked me to call her back. I didn't know either, but it couldn't hurt to have another opinion, so I quickly dialed her number.

"Hello, Mrs. Parker," came the cheerful answer when I explained who I was. "We received your husband's referral information a few weeks ago. Have you decided if you'd like one of our surgeons to review it?"

Every muscle in my body contracted, and my head began to pound. How could she sound so calm? Didn't she realize the world was falling apart and she had helped speed it along by not processing the referral? Why did everything have to be so complicated, and why did all the professionals not seem the slightest bit bothered by any of it?

I savored the image of reaching through the phone and ripping her head off while I debated how loudly I should scream. I knew that would not help Blaine, so instead I took a deep breath and just said, "Yes, please send the information to the surgeon." It wasn't nearly as satisfying as my dream of separating her head from her body, but it got things rolling once again.

My heart was pounding through my chest as I shoved my phone into my pocket and stepped outside for some air. "*Why* is this happening, and *why* doesn't anyone care?" I said aloud to God as I dropped onto the step. A warm breeze caressed my skin, and a pair of mourning doves cooed to each other in the trees near our deck. I took a deep breath and felt my tense muscles relax a bit but had no answer to my questions.

I closed my eyes and tilted my face up toward the sun, trying to wrap my head around the way the scheduler had been so calm. Where was her sense of panic? She had to understand that time was critical, that the most important person in my world could die if he wasn't treated quickly. If I worked in a cancer hospital, I'd be panicked all the time.

My shoulders slumped and I opened my eyes as the truth settled over me. If I worked in a cancer hospital, I wouldn't be panicked because I would be in contact with hundreds of patients a week in the exact same situation. While cancer was new and terrifying to me, to the people working in the hospitals, it was normal. They couldn't do their jobs if they got upset about every single patient. I needed them to be calm and collected so they could get Blaine the treatment he needed. I had to learn to be patient and to trust the professionals to do their jobs.

The scheduler called first thing the next morning. "Dr. Knobloch reviewed your husband's MRI images, and she is very concerned. She would like you both to come here as soon as possible."

My body suddenly felt heavier, and I sank into the couch. Disappointment washed over me, and I realized I had been hoping she would say it all looked fine. "What exactly does she want to do if we come?" I squeaked out.

"She wants to schedule a biopsy of the mass, as well as a more detailed MRI of Blaine's arm and a CT scan of his chest and abdomen, among other smaller tests."

I was silent for a minute as I willed my brain to understand what she was saying. Finally, it started working again, and I asked, "How long will all of that take?"

"Oh, we can get those all scheduled within a day or two of each other, but Dr. Knobloch needs you to stay in Houston for a week in case other tests are needed and so you will be available to meet with whatever doctors are necessary." She paused for a moment before dropping the final blow. "She says you need to come by next week."

I was glad I was sitting down as I was pretty sure my legs wouldn't have held me up. "How soon do you need to know our plans?"

"Soon."

I promised to let her know quickly and hung up to call Blaine. Next week he was scheduled to have surgery in St. Louis. Should we proceed with that plan and potentially be done with the whole ordeal, or should we waste time doing more tests? We didn't know what to do, so we prayed. We prayed and prayed and prayed. Compared to going all the way to Houston, it seemed so simple to just get Lumpy taken care of in St. Louis. How could we possibly stay in Houston for an entire week and then go back to have it removed?

We just wanted this to be over, to get our lives back, but I still had this nagging feeling that Trinity was not the right choice. Finally, I told Blaine I thought we needed to go to Houston. "If somehow this thing goes south, I don't want to have to live with the fact that we did the cheapest thing." He agreed, and the next day I called and canceled his surgery at Trinity. They acted like I had lost my mind. I wasn't 100 percent sure that I hadn't, but I did it anyway.

Now we were scrambling to make plans. I was terrified to spend any money we didn't absolutely have to but learned that flights were actually available from Springfield to Houston for less money than it would cost us to drive. I quickly booked the tickets and breathed a sigh of relief. One task was done!

Now we needed a place to stay. MD Anderson's website contains a long list of hotels that offer discounts for their patients, but each hotel had different amenities and different rates, and it was completely overwhelming to me. I was still having trouble thinking clearly, and this list was simply more than I could handle. After staring at it for an hour, I finally gave up and called one of my sisters. I asked her to choose one for us. I told her what we needed as far as shuttles and breakfast and asked her to process all the information and just make the decision for me.

She called back a few hours later with her top three recommendations ... and told me she and her husband were going to pay for it. I sat there silently for a few moments trying to process what she had said and then thankfully accepted. It was the first time we took money from anyone, and I think a little part of me died. I felt embarrassed, but I also felt loved. I felt overwhelmed with my need, but I also felt overwhelmed with God's provision. I felt a million things all at once. Again, with my sludge-filled mind, I just couldn't quite process any of it, so I didn't. I just said, "Thank you," and moved on. There was no choice but to keep moving forward, to do the next thing. This mentality was going to become my new way of life, but sitting in my office on the phone with my sister was the first real sense that I just had to take the next step, I had to keep moving forward, no matter how uncomfortable or hard it was. She actually called and made the hotel reservation for me. One more task was done!

We took care of all the final little details. Thankfully, Kaia was still home. She had been living on her own for the last year, and I felt better knowing she was there. Kaci and Kamryn are mature and competent, but somehow having the oldest one at home made me feel safer. Kaci was still in her brace and on crutches but was more mobile by this time, and everyone was more comfortable with her needs. Kamryn had finished her school year. Blaine and I informed our employers we would be gone, and I stocked the girls up with groceries. The day of our flight arrived much too quickly and somehow too slowly at the same time. Kaia drove us all to the airport. Blaine and I hugged the girls goodbye and walked in having absolutely no idea how different we would be when we walked back through those doors a week later.

Chapter 8

The flight was uneventful, and we easily found an Uber and checked into the hotel. We went down for breakfast the next morning and were surprised by the number of people there. I began this sick game in my head of trying to guess who was a cancer patient and who wasn't. I wondered if anyone could tell Blaine had cancer. Some of the people would come and go over the next week, but some stayed, and it was a little bit comforting to see them every day, like we were in the same club. It was a club no one wanted to be in but still encouraging not to feel totally alone.

The next day was Saturday, and Blaine was scheduled for a COVID test. The hotel shuttle drove us, along with some other people, right to the building. It wasn't in the main part of the hospital, just one of the many that comprised the MD Anderson campus. Even though I had been there before with my friend, I was completely overwhelmed with the size of the facility. There were so many buildings! It made Trinity Hospital look tiny. It seems even bigger because it is in the same area as multiple other large hospitals. I knew I was going to need to learn my way around, but I couldn't fathom actually being able to do that.

Because of the COVID pandemic, only patients were allowed to go inside. I found a bench and waited while Blaine went to have his test done. He had never had a COVID test before, and I was a little concerned for him. I needn't have worried. He came out twenty minutes later just fine. He said he had found the room without any problems and had actually *laughed* when they put the stick up his nose! The shuttle driver came back to pick us up, and all that was left to do for the next couple of days was to wait to make sure his test was negative.

As expected, Blaine did not have COVID, and Monday found us back at the hospital for the day of tests. Houston in the summer is approximately the same temperature as the surface of the sun, but I was able to find a spot in the shade and really wasn't too uncomfortable. Blaine was scheduled for blood tests, an EKG, a CT scan of his chest and abdomen, an MRI of his arm, and a biopsy of Lumpy. Between tests he came back to visit with me.

Eventually, someone told him about a space inside another part of the hospital which had been designated for companions, and we went to find it. We walked through the automatic sliding doors and deliciously cool air swept over us. I glanced around as people in front of us went through the COVID screening. Two-story windows flooded the area with sunlight. Beautiful chandeliers hung from the ceiling, and big, soft chairs welcomed people to stop and rest. Employees bustled by while patients slogged their way past us on to their next appointments.

Finally, it was our turn. We washed our hands with the sanitizer, and then the screener handed us fresh masks. "Are you here for an appointment?"

"I am," Blaine answered.

"Okay." He glanced at me. "You will need to stay in our companion waiting area." He nodded his head toward a collection of chairs surrounded by a small cord. "You are not allowed outside of the designated area." He turned to Blaine. "And you are not allowed inside it." Blaine and I glanced at each other and smiled under our masks. Thank goodness there was a cord! Surely the COVID germs knew they had to stay inside! The screener went through his list of questions to confirm we were most likely safe to enter and then let us pass. Blaine leaned over the cord and kissed me and then went on to his next appointment while I settled down in one of the comfortable chairs, treasuring the cool air.

One of Blaine's appointments that day was with his surgeon, Dr. Knobloch. Unlike Trinity Hospital, MD Anderson had assigned a surgeon who specializes exclusively in soft tissue sarcomas of the extremities. Blaine put me on speakerphone so I could hear what she had to say and ask questions. By this point in the pandemic, the doctors were used to this, and Dr. Knobloch and her assistant made me feel comfortable, like this was a totally normal way to do things. I liked her immediately. She was warm and friendly and seemed completely confident in her ability to get rid of Lumpy. "I still need to see the images from our stronger machine, but I have studied your MRI results from Springfield, and it looks like the tumor is well encapsulated. It's not branching out into your other tissues, and it should be easy to get out."

I breathed a sigh of relief. Finally, some good news! Unfortunately, she went on. "You will need to stay in Houston for three weeks for the surgery."

I waited for Blaine to say something, but he was silent, so I plunged in. "I don't understand. I thought it was going to be easy to get out. The hospital in St. Louis only needed him to stay overnight."

"Really? We must do things very differently. We'll need Blaine to be in town for about a week before surgery to undergo final tests and prep work. Then after the surgery he will stay in the hospital for five days. After he is released, he will need to remain in town for another week just to make sure there are no complications. It will be easy to get the tumor out, but it's still a complicated surgery."

I swallowed hard and fought down the panic rising in my chest. *Three weeks!* How on earth were we going to make that work? We had jobs and kids at home. Three weeks was an awfully long time to be gone.

Blaine finally spoke up. "How soon will you be able to do the surgery?"

"That depends. After all the results of today's tests are in, you will meet with a radiation oncologist and a medical oncologist." She paused for a moment. She knew she was about to deliver hard news. "If chemotherapy is recommended, you will be able to receive that at home, but if you need radiation, you will have to stay in Houston for a few more weeks before the surgery."

Blaine and I sat in stunned silence. The panic that had been trying to take over with the idea of staying in Houston for three weeks burst past my fragile control, but I quickly shoved it back down. Surely, he would not need radiation. We'd find a way to deal with the three weeks. It couldn't possibly be worse than that. Dr. Knobloch wrapped up the appointment, and Blaine made his way back to the waiting area. Neither of us mentioned the radiation issue again.

The schedulers had done an amazing job arranging all of his appointments and even left a small break for lunch. This was important because after a certain time, Blaine was not allowed to eat so he could have contrast dye for the CT scan. On paper, this looked like a great plan. Unfortunately, every single department was running behind schedule, some of them significantly behind. We were told later that pre-COVID this never would have happened, but it was certainly an issue now. Each department was able to adjust accordingly, but it meant we missed our much-needed lunch break, and we ended up going more than twelve hours without food.

I could have easily eaten while Blaine was undergoing his tests, but I had this idea that if he was suffering, I should too. This was not smart. In the coming months, I would learn it was critical to take care of myself so I could be ready to help him as much as possible. I wasn't helping anyone by not eating.

Finally, he was finished with everything. We called the hotel shuttle driver who quickly came to pick us up. We ordered a pizza on the way back and completely devoured it as soon as we got to our room.

As unpleasant as the day had been, the next few days were worse. We had to wait for the results of the CT scan to see if the cancer had spread to other parts of his body. This is the main concern with sarcomas. We knew Lumpy would be easy to remove from Blaine's arm, but if it had spread to other places, we were looking at a much more dire situation. So much time had passed since he had first felt the tiny lump in his arm; there had certainly been time for it to spread. Blaine seemed to be totally calm. I was in the bathroom ten times a day. We didn't know when they would call with the results, and every time his phone rang, my heart would beat uncontrollably and I had trouble catching my breath. It only took a few days for the results to come in, but it felt like months. They were the longest days of my life.

Finally, one morning Blaine's phone rang, and we could tell it was the surgeon's office. Blaine put it on speaker, and we sat down to hear the news.

"I have good news for you, Mr. and Mrs. Parker!" My muscles that had been clenched for the last week slowly relaxed as her words sunk in. "There are no signs of any metastases anywhere else in your body. That is a very good thing! However, the biopsy did show that you have a very high-grade undifferentiated sarcoma." I had no idea what those words meant, but, thankfully, she went on to explain. "High-grade" meant it was growing very quickly, and "undifferentiated" meant its cells were not a specific type and thus were likely to spread even faster than typical cancer cells. Blaine was scheduled to meet with the radiation and medical oncologists the next day. We needed to make a plan and get Lumpy out of him as soon as possible.

Chapter 9

The next morning I found myself once again sitting on a bench near the shockingly busy street in front of the hospital. I knew I would feel uncomfortable having conversations with the doctors where everyone around me could hear, so we decided I would stay outside. Blaine went in for his appointment, and I settled down to wait.

I didn't have to wait long. Blaine was already learning his way around the giant hospital quite well. He went right to the department and was quickly led back for his appointment. Soon Dr. Gancio, the radiation oncologist, and her resident came in. They introduced themselves to Blaine and said hello to me through the phone. They were personable and professional and I immediately liked them both. "We've gone over all of your results. We're sorry you're having to deal with this, but we do feel confident that our radiation protocol will be very effective in killing the cancer cells."

"I want to do the surgery first. Then, if it's decided I still need radiation, we can deal with that afterward," Blaine informed them.

"I'm afraid that would be a very dangerous mistake," Dr. Gancio replied. "Doing the radiation first is essential to ensure any cancer cells in the area are killed. If they do the surgery before killing the surrounding cells, the cancer will likely be dispersed through your entire body.

My hands began to tremble. "That is exactly what the surgeon at Trinity[5] planned to do."

Both doctors gasped. "That would have been extremely hazardous. Under no circumstances should a high-grade sarcoma be excised without killing the surrounding cells with radiation first."

The trembling in my hands continued and my mouth went dry. We had come so close to having Lumpy taken care of at Trinity. Their plan had made sense to us, and getting it just cut off was what we really wanted to do. What if we had proceeded with that plan? It became crystal clear at that moment why I had felt so unsettled about seeking treatment at a perfectly respectable and logical hospital. God clearly was guiding us. It had seemed like He wasn't really answering our prayers, but He obviously was, and I am so thankful He made sure we ended up where we needed to be.

Dr. Gancio went on to cheerfully tell us that Blaine only needed five weeks of daily radiation treatments.

Wait! What? *Five* weeks? Again, I was sitting by the side of a busy road. Surely I had misheard her! "I'm sorry. Can you repeat that? How many weeks does he need?"

"Five weeks. He'll come in every weekday for five weeks, a total of just twenty-five treatments."

"Can we just have that done at home? You could tell the hospital there how you want it done and they could just do it?" By this point, I had read everything I could find about MD Anderson, and I knew they often prescribed protocols and patients were able to have those carried out in their hometowns.

"I'm sorry. The radiation treatments really must be administered here at our facility. Now, if it is recommended that he receive chemotherapy, that can be done at home."

"Why does the radiation have to be done here?" Blaine asked.

At this point, Dr. Gancio seemed embarrassed and uncomfortable. Finally, she said, "It is absolutely imperative that the radiation be given in the exactly correct way. Technique is critically important and . . . well . . . we are simply the best. Our staff are very highly trained, and our equipment is the absolute top in the industry. If the radiation is not given exactly perfectly, it will not be as effective. It really must be done here."

I don't know how you make a statement like this and not come off sounding arrogant, but she didn't. She sounded honest.

"The good news is that radiation is easy for the patient. You may feel a little more tired toward the end, and your skin may get a little red, but you will otherwise feel fine. The treatment will take approximately fifteen minutes a day, but other than that, you will be free to work or do whatever you want."

"Will he be able to drive?"

"Certainly. He will feel fine."

By this point, my mind was racing. I still wasn't sure how we were going to swing being in Houston for three weeks for the surgery. Now we were going to have to be here for *five additional weeks*? Slowly I remembered she said Blaine would feel fine. Maybe I didn't actually need to be here with him the whole time. That wasn't ideal, but we obviously couldn't leave the girls for eight weeks. Blaine had worked from home some during the COVID shutdown. Maybe he could just bring his computer with him and work here after his treatment sessions. I could stay home with the girls and just fly down for a weekend or two. My mind was still reeling, but I started to feel a little better. It was going to be hard, but we would figure out a way to make it work. Dr. Gancio answered a few more questions and told Blaine she was looking forward to seeing him again, and he left for his next appointment.

Soon, Blaine was in the medical oncologist's office, and Dr. Baldyga and her assistant came in to meet him. She got right to the point. "Mr. Parker, you have a very high-grade sarcoma, but with chemotherapy, I am confident I can cure you."

Despite the heat, my body went cold. Did she really say Blaine needed chemotherapy? That made no sense. There was no sign of metastases. The surgeon was confident she could remove Lumpy, and now the radiation oncologist was confident she could kill any cancer cells that might be in the area. Why on earth would he need chemotherapy on top of that?

I could tell Blaine was just as shocked as I was. "Why would I need chemotherapy if the tumor is just on my arm, and they can cut it out?"

"Because sarcomas are very sneaky and very aggressive, and yours in particular is growing very quickly. There are probably microscopic sarcoma cells throughout your body that are simply too small now to show on the MRI. We will use the chemotherapy to kill them before they have a chance to come together and form more tumors."

That sort of made sense to me, but the idea of Blaine going through chemotherapy made me sick to my stomach. I had witnessed first-hand its horrors when his mother had been sick. I decided then I would never do that, or advise anyone I loved to do that, but suddenly here we were, facing the decision of whether the person I loved most in the world would have to endure it. The one comfort I had was that I knew cancer treatment had come a long way in the twenty years since Blaine's mom's experience. Surely it wouldn't be as hard on him as it had been on his mother.

While all of this was racing through my mind, Dr. Baldyga continued. "The chemotherapy treatment will take four-and-a-half months, then you will receive radiation, then they will do the surgery."

She had an unfamiliar accent, and I was sitting next to the street listening on a phone. Surely she hadn't said four-and-a-half months! "Excuse me," I said, "Could you please repeat that?"

"The chemotherapy treatment will take four-and-a-half months . . ." I stopped listening. I was doing math in my head while trying to keep my brain from exploding. We could have had Lumpy removed by now, but instead they were recommending keeping it in for six more months?

"So, he would receive the chemo treatments at home and then return here for the radiation and surgery, right?"

"Oh no! The chemo treatments will have to be administered here."

At this point, I am sure my brain is actually exploding. "What? Why? We were told if he had to have chemo, he could do that at home."

"Who told you that?"

"Everyone. Literally everyone we spoke to said if he needed chemo, he could do that at home."

"They should not have told you that. That is not true. The chemotherapy recommended for sarcomas is so very strong that regular hospitals do not know how to use it. They are not prepared for the side effects, and I cannot assure his safety if he is not here."

I let that piece of information sink in. *The chemotherapy recommended for sarcomas is so very strong that regular hospitals do not know how to use it . . . cannot assure his safety . . .* My brain was definitely exploding. The image of Blaine finding me in a gooey puddle by the side of the street flashes through my mind.

I managed to pull myself together. "This seems pretty extreme considering there are no actual signs of metastases, and they can easily remove the tumor that we know is there."

"The five-year life expectancy for a patient with sarcoma who doesn't do chemotherapy is only 65 percent." Honestly, I had read this statistic, but somehow I had assumed it was wrong. Hearing the words come from one of the top oncologists in the country was horrifying.

She went on to say that while he would need to receive all of his treatments in Houston, at some point he would be able to go home for a bit in between the cycles. It was all so confusing. My mind was still completely reeling at the news, and I knew nothing really about chemotherapy. What was a "cycle"? Dr. Baldyga's accent, the noise from the street traffic, and the unbearable heat were certainly not helping.

Blaine told her he was not sure what he wanted to do; she stressed that he needed to make a decision quickly, and he left. We went back to the hotel, packed our bags, and headed for the airport. I could not wait to see our girls. Our whole world had been turned upside down, and I wanted nothing more than to wrap my arms around our children and pretend everything was normal. Unfortunately, that was not the case, and we couldn't ignore the fact that we now had to make the most important decision of our lives.

Chapter 10

Posted all over the hospital and included in the welcome packet we had been given was information on how to access our patient advocate if we had any issues with our care. It wasn't necessarily that we had an issue with his care, but we were so surprised Dr. Baldyga would think Blaine needed chemotherapy. We had been told one of the best things about MD Anderson was that all of the medical recommendations were made by a team of doctors. We really wanted to know someone else had looked at his information and agreed he needed the treatment Dr. Baldyga was recommending. We weren't angry with her. It wasn't that we thought she had done anything wrong. We simply wanted a second opinion. We contacted our assigned patient advocate and explained the situation.

Three days later we found ourselves on a conference call with the patient advocate and Dr. Baldyga, who had been told we were unhappy with her care. As far as we knew, no other doctor had been given Blaine's information to review[6], and now his assigned oncologist thought we didn't like her. This was absolutely not what we were hoping for. She was very sweet on the phone and once again explained why she thought Blaine needed the prescribed treatment. She reiterated that his five-year life expectancy without chemotherapy was not good.

The one helpful thing about this conversation is that we were able to get more detailed information about what his schedule would look like. Dr. Baldyga explained that Blaine's chemotherapy cycles would be three weeks. Each of the first four days of the cycle, he would come to the hospital for an IV infusion of one chemotherapy drug (ifosfamide), and he would go home with a pump hooked to him for a twenty-four-hour infusion of another type (doxorubicin), as well as a bag of a medicine called mesna that would protect his bladder from the doxorubicin. Then he would have two weeks to rest before beginning the next cycle. Because of the strength of those particular drugs and the dosages he would be receiving, they absolutely must be administered at MD Anderson. Other clinicians would not know how to safely manage them or be prepared to handle the potential side effects. Blaine would need to stay in Houston for the entire first cycle (three weeks) and through the administration of the second round of chemo, but then should be safe to come home for the resting two weeks. He could go back and forth for each cycle after that for a total of six cycles, approximately four-and-a-half months.

We told Dr. Baldyga we would need to pray about it, and she stressed that we needed to make a decision quickly so Lumpy did not have time to spread. We hung up the phone and sat there staring at each other. We were now facing an impossible decision. For the next five days, all of my thoughts centered on what he should do. I had to work, and I had to continue managing our family, but I felt like it all faded to the background. I was going through the motions of functioning normally, but in reality, my brain was completely fixated on whether or not Blaine should take the chemotherapy treatments.

Our limited experience with chemo had not been good. In my early twenties, I had watched a friend's husband beat cancer, but then die from the effects of the chemotherapy treatment he had taken. We had both watched Blaine's mom suffer tremendously from chemotherapy only to die anyway. Then just a few years earlier, we had a dear friend who was receiving chemotherapy die suddenly from a mouth sore because the chemo, which had caused the mouth sore, had knocked her white count so low she was not able to fight the infection. This haunted me, and I thought about her constantly. She had gone from almost fine to dead with no warning—from a mouth sore. Should we risk this happening to Blaine when there was no evidence at all there were any cancer cells anywhere besides his arm? Should we risk the chance there were cancer cells inside him and they would spread and kill him because he hadn't done the treatment? Both choices were terrifying.

At this point, we knew we needed help. We needed all the prayer support we could get. Blaine spent an agonizing Sunday afternoon calling various family members. It was a long, emotional day, and even though I didn't do anything, I was completely worn out by the time he was done.

After those closest to him all knew, I posted the news on Facebook, and just like that, the word was officially out. Honestly, this was a relief. We no longer had to try to remember who knew and who didn't, and we didn't have to pretend everything was fine. Plus, within a few hours hundreds of people had told us they would be praying. This was a huge shift for us. Knowing so many people cared and would be supporting us through whatever happened gave us hope we would make it.

We prayed more in those five days than ever before in our lives. We needed wisdom. We had absolutely no idea what to do. We knew that any healing Blaine might receive would completely be from God, but we had no idea how He planned to achieve that or which direction that meant we should take. There were two people in particular whose opinions we sought. One had lost her husband recently to a brain tumor; the other was in the midst of fighting colon cancer. Interestingly, those two refused to tell us. They did listen for hours to my rambling thoughts and did their best to help me sort those out, but they never just told me what they thought we should do. They knew how much influence they would have over us, but they also knew it had to be our decision. It's such a fine line to share your knowledge without pushing someone toward your position, and they had both mastered this skill beautifully.

Soon we knew what we should do. Blaine should not take the chemo. God was the ultimate healer. If He wanted Blaine to be healed, He could certainly do it without our letting the doctors put poison into his body. It was completely illogical to take a chance of killing him with the chemo when there was no evidence there were any extra sarcoma cells inside him. It just made sense to do the radiation and then get Lumpy out of him as quickly as possible. We would contact Dr. Baldyga in the morning and tell her.

The next morning, we woke up and knew what we should do. Blaine *should* take the chemo. God had given people the intelligence to know how to use chemotherapy to kill cancer. It just made sense to use that to our advantage. It was completely illogical to take a chance of leaving any random sarcoma cells inside him that could potentially kill him. He was young and healthy. If we waited until the cancer had a chance to move to his lungs, he might not be healthy enough to withstand the necessary treatment. Obviously, we needed to do it now. What had we been thinking the day before?

This process repeated itself over and over and over. Multiple times a day our thinking completely shifted. We agreed that ultimately the decision had to be Blaine's, but he always wanted to know my opinion. Surprisingly, through all the many, many twists, we were always on the same page at the same time. I'm so thankful for this, but we were exhausted and frustrated. We were begging God for direction but getting nothing. I was not sure if He wasn't answering or if I was just too dense to understand Him, but either way, we had no clue what we should do.

We were both confident God had led us to MD Anderson, and ultimately we just decided it didn't make sense to seek treatment eleven hours away because we felt they had the best doctors, and then not follow their advice. There was never any sort of clear spiritual revelation that he needed the chemo, and we never had any sort of huge mental relief that we had made the right decision. It was really simply a matter of looking at all the pros and cons and making a choice. We needed to trust the people who knew more than we did. We messaged Dr. Baldyga that Blaine would take the chemo, and we went to bed. Neither of us felt good about the decision, but at least we didn't have to keep thinking about it.

Chapter 11

The very next day we received a message that all of Blaine's initial appointments to start the chemo had been scheduled. We had approximately thirty hours before we needed to leave for a month in Texas. *Thirty hours*! We had no place to stay; we had no transportation, and Kaci and Kamryn would be home by themselves for weeks, even though Kaci had barely turned eighteen. Kaia was set to go back to school so she could train with her team and get the final rehab she needed for her elbow. Thankfully, Kaci had just been taken off crutches, but she still had physical therapy appointments and had started a new job. Kamryn's fifteenth birthday would happen while we were gone. I had thirty hours to manufacture a workable plan and zero clue how to do that.

Thankfully, God was not surprised by any of this and had already worked it out. That morning my phone buzzed, and I looked down to discover our friend, Amanda, was calling. After asking how we were holding up, she dove right in. "A friend from high school is now a pastor in Houston. I called him to see if he had any idea where you could stay while you're there. It turns out his church operates a ministry that provides free housing for patients coming to the area for medical care. He's setting everything up for you. You just need to call them."

Tears stung my eyes as I sank into my chair. Other than leaving the girls alone, my biggest worry was where we would stay for a whole month in Texas. I quickly called the number Amanda had given and spoke with the director of Mercy House Ministries. She let me know arrangements had been made for us to stay in one of their houses with two other cancer patients and their caregivers for the entire time we were there—for free! This was so above and beyond anything I could have hoped for! The entire situation was so shocking and scary to me, but God had arranged the solution years earlier.

Then Kaia came to us and announced she had decided to stay home through the month of July. We were so touched by this! We knew her best chance of making the lineup for the next season depended on getting back to work with the trainers who knew best how to strengthen her elbow and the coaches who made the decision on who competed and who didn't. She had dreamed for years of competing in college, and she was aware the decision to stay home another month might affect her ability to do that, but she knew her family needed her, and she put us first. She could stay until we came home in four weeks, and then I would take her back. It certainly wasn't ideal, but it would work. I wrapped her in a bear hug and closed my eyes so I could savor the moment. I missed her so much when she was at school. I couldn't believe she was finally home, and I was going to miss out on my time with her.

Soon the phone rang. It was my friend, Debbie. "How are you holding up?"

I breathed out an awkward laugh. I never knew how I should answer that question. "I'm doing okay," I lied.

"I was just wondering if you might want to take Faith's car to Texas." I sucked in my breath. Our car situation was a big problem. One of our cars was on its last legs. It didn't seem wise to take it on a long trip, nor did it seem wise to leave our teenage girls home alone with it while we took our good car. "It's just sitting here. I know she'd love for you to use it."

"We'll be gone for four weeks."

"I know. That's fine. Use it as long as you need it!"

I gushed out my thanks and sank back into my chair. We had met Debbie fifteen years earlier when Kaia started taking gymnastics classes at her gym.

Debbie's daughter, Faith, had left recently to be a missionary in a foreign country. While she was ministering to the people there, she would also minister to us. I know the timing of her trip and our need for a car was not a coincidence. In a matter of maybe twenty minutes, our three biggest needs had been resolved.

It might have been good that we had such little notice before we had to leave, as it didn't allow much time to dwell on how scared and sad we were. Weirdly though, our dogs seemed to know, and they stayed pretty much glued to me the entire time before we left. I hadn't even wanted to get them, but now I loved them so much! I would really miss them while we were gone.

Many friends stopped by to see us that day and to remind us we were loved. They promised to pray for us and to make sure the girls had what they needed. Some gave us cash, gift cards, or things to keep me entertained and distracted. One friend gave me some words of wisdom that would completely change my outlook. We were standing on our front porch as they were getting ready to leave, and I was whining about how scary it was that the chemo they were going to give Blaine was so strong that other hospitals would not be able to handle it.

"That's awesome," he said.

I was totally taken aback. "What do you mean it's awesome?"

"If you're going to war, you don't want to take Switzerland. You want the strongest army you can find. Blaine is going into battle, and they're arming him with the very strongest defense possible. That's totally awesome!"

This was such a huge moment for me! He was right! We were going into a battle, and I wanted Blaine equipped to fight with everything possible. It made no sense to just throw a little bit of medicine at it. He needed the big guns, and we were on our way to get them!

Early the next morning, we hugged the girls goodbye and started the eleven-hour trip. It was so bizarre to think that we wouldn't be back for a whole month! All of us had a busy day coming up. While Blaine and I would spend the day in the car, Kaia was flying to Iowa for a couple of days, Kaci had an appointment to see her surgeon in Kansas, and Kamryn would be spending the day at a friend's house. We would all be in different states! For a momma who really likes all of her family to be together, this made me a little crazy, but I did my best not to think about it.

The drive to Houston was long, but, thankfully, uneventful. Blaine drove the whole way. A friend had taken Kaci to her appointment, and they kept me updated. Her hip was healing exactly as expected, so that was good news. Kaia's plane was a little delayed taking off from Springfield, but that was no big deal. She had never flown anywhere by herself, but she was very competent and independent, and I wasn't worried about her. Kamryn was having a great time at her friend's house, and I was so thankful she had something to distract her. Unfortunately, we arrived in Houston right at rush hour. I grew up in a town with only one blinking red light, and being in a lot of traffic is something I hate. Houston is the fourth most densely populated city in the country, so the traffic is always bad. This would be an ongoing issue for me, and starting off on the giant highway downtown at rush hour was not a good plan, but I survived.

I received a text while we were driving saying the house we had been assigned to stay in was having problems with the air conditioner. The Mercy House director apologized but said we would need to go to a different location until it could be fixed. We didn't care in the slightest; we were just so thankful we had a place to stay! When we arrived at the new house, Lydia, the woman from the church who managed it, met us and showed us around.

"You'll actually be the only ones in the house tonight, but another couple is scheduled to arrive tomorrow. Two more couples will come on Monday, so I'm afraid you won't be able to stay here, but surely the AC will be fixed in the other house by then." She led us to the kitchen and showed us where to find everything we might need. She had even stocked the kitchen with basic food. We were all set.

We settled in and were just about to go to bed when Kaia called. "Hi, Sweetie! I thought you'd be in the air by now."

"I missed my connecting flight. I'm not sure what to do."

My heart sank. The idea of my "baby" being stuck alone on the other side of the country made me sick to my stomach, and there was nothing I could do to help her. Eventually she was able to get on a flight that would get her reasonably close to her destination, and a friend agreed to pick her up in the middle of the night. It all worked out fine, but the fact that it was our first day away and we had already faced a situation in which one of our girls needed us and we were too far away to help them was unsettling. The pit in my stomach gnawed angrily as I finally climbed into bed, but there was nothing I could do but ignore it and force myself to go to sleep. I was so anxious to get the next few weeks over with and back to our normal lives.

Chapter 12

The next two days were a whirlwind of appointments and tests. In between these, we attended a mandatory chemo class where a nurse taught the basics of how chemotherapy works, ways to make the process easier, and signs to watch for that indicate the patient must be taken to the emergency room. While all of us were dealing with different types of protocols and different types of cancer, the basic fundamental issues of surviving chemotherapy are the same.

I took notes furiously. I was overwhelmed with the fact that Blaine's comfort over the next few weeks, and possibly whether he lived or died, depended somewhat on how well I was able to follow the directions and information I was being given. The fact that we would be totally alone through this, there would be no one around to help me remember or to help with his care, was terrifying. I wrote down everything. I underlined and highlighted and drew circles around the most important parts. I was determined to be the best caregiver possible but was pretty sure I was going to fail.

I was actually looking forward to this class. I assumed we would meet people who were going through our exact circumstances and instantly become fast friends. That did not happen. While everyone was friendly, each person, even the ones who had clearly been through chemotherapy treatments before, looked stunned and too scared to chat. I think everyone worries their whole life that they or someone they love are going to get cancer, but when it happens, it's so hard to actually believe. You draw into yourself and are only focused on surviving it. Part of me totally felt this, but I also desperately needed to be with other people who would get what we were dealing with.

One of the procedures Blaine had during this time was the placement of his CVC (central venous catheter). The CVC is a flexible tube that is placed directly into a vein. Blaine's CVC went into his chest and had two lines, called lumens, that hung down outside his skin. One of these had a white cap and the other an orange cap, so each line could be identified. These could be connected to IV lines so the chemo and other medicines could be administered without having to stick him each time. His blood could also be drawn directly through the lumens to check his labs. Although he was pretty sore for the next day or so, eventually he wouldn't even notice it, and he was so happy he didn't have to be poked over and over!

Although we were very grateful for the CVC line, it came with one serious drawback: the constant risk of infection. If any bacteria found its way into the tube directly into his chest, it could kill him quickly. Each of the lines had to be flushed daily and completely replaced every week. It was so critical this be done correctly that the caregivers had to take a mandatory class and then demonstrate their ability to correctly care for it before the CVC could be used. I was not concerned about this. I have a degree in sports medicine and had taught first aid courses for years. How hard could it be?

The class was filled with different people than those who had been in our chemotherapy class, a testament to just how many patients were at MD Anderson. They showed us a video and then had us practice on the lumens they provided. There was actually quite a bit to remember, and the teacher drilled into us the crucial importance that each step be followed precisely or we could kill our loved one. (No pressure!). She mentioned there was also a video online showing how to replace the lumens if we would not be close to the hospital and needed to do that at home.

The next day Blaine and I went to the vascular department for my appointed time to demonstrate I could care for his CVC. A different nurse was in charge of determining whether or not I was competent to clean it. I was nervous but did okay. Then she asked if we would be going home. "Yes!" I announced a little too enthusiastically.

"So you will need to replace the tubing." My confidence vanished. Thankfully, I had watched the video on how to change it, but I hadn't really given it much thought. I was concentrating on taking things one day at a time, and my needing to switch out the tubing was close to thirty days away. "Show me how to replace the tubing safely," she said.

I tried to demonstrate what I remembered from the video, but it was painfully clear I had no clue what I was doing. She, somewhat patiently, guided me through. It all felt so awkward! I had watched nurses handle similar tasks like it was the most natural thing in the world, but I felt so clumsy. After going through it a couple of times, with repeated sighs of frustration from both of us, she either finally determined I had a chance of not killing my husband, or she just got tired of dealing with me and eventually signed the paperwork and let me go. I walked into the hall and called my nurse friend who promised to change it for me when we were home. I was not used to being incompetent. A sense this would not be the last time I would feel this way hung over me, but at least I had found a solution for this particular problem.

We went back to the house and discovered our housemates had arrived. Bradley and Elesha were from Mississippi, and we loved them immediately. Bradley had been fighting esophageal cancer for years and had come to MD Anderson to start a promising new clinical trial. In addition to being the friends I was seeking who were facing the same situation, they provided the extra bonus of experience and were a fantastic source of information and guidance. Elesha was also an Alabama football fan, so she and Blaine bonded immediately! We enjoyed dinner together that evening, and because they didn't have a car with them, we were able to help them get to appointments and run errands. They weren't in town long, but we quickly built a relationship that would last.

The next day as I was walking through the hospital, Lydia called. She asked how things were going and then broke the news I didn't want to hear. "We have a problem. The air conditioner is still not fixed at the other house, and the scheduled guests are going to arrive in the morning. You're going to have to move out."

I stopped right in the middle of the busy hallway and then slumped against the wall and pressed my hand to my temple, attempting to relieve the stabbing pain that had started. I was proud of how I was holding myself together, but one more problem might undo me.

"Don't panic!" she went on as if she could see me. "My husband and I have a small pool house in our backyard that we sometimes use for patients if all the mercy houses are full. You and Blaine are welcome to stay there until the other house is ready."

I took a deep breath and the stabbing pain disappeared. I thanked her profusely and then went to find Blaine. We couldn't have cared less where we stayed. We were just so thankful to have a roof over our heads. As soon as his appointments were done for the day, we quickly packed up our stuff and drove to our new home.

Although we were not far from the place we had been staying, the further we drove, the bigger the houses became. When we pulled onto our new street, we gasped. Hundred-year-old live oaks stood guard over homes so luxurious and meticulously landscaped, I feared we, in our borrowed Kia Soul, wouldn't be allowed to enter. We pulled into Lydia's drive, and she came out to meet us. She gave us a remote to open the gate and told us her only real rule was that we always ensure the gate was closed so her dogs would not get out. Dogs?

I perked up at that but didn't have time to process what she had said because we soon walked around the corner, and I saw where we would be staying. I hoped Lydia didn't see my mouth falling open, but it couldn't be helped. Beautiful trees and wildflowers bounded the edges of the yard, and butterflies and birds flitted around in the sun. Blue water in a tiled pool and hot tub invited us to relax in the center of the yard. As we walked a little further, I heard babbling and looked over to see water rushing over large rocks into a quiet pool below. I could not wait to sit next to the ferns and feel the mist on my face. A sense of peace swept over me, and even the air felt lighter. We heard a ruckus and turned to see mounds of curly white fur rushing to greet us. Lily, Daisy, and Holly were Lydia's "kids," and I knew I was going to love them.

I couldn't stop smiling as I soaked it all in. We were minutes from the largest cancer hospital in one of the largest cities in the country, and we were surrounded by trees, flowers, and wildlife. I was raised in the country, and even in the best of times, I crave nature and quiet. Water is particularly comforting to me, and God had even provided a waterfall. Then, just to top it off a little more, He had even sent dogs! I was afraid I might wake up and discover I had been dreaming, but it was all real. After a few days, Lydia and her husband decided we could just stay as long as we were in town. There could not have been a better place for us![7]

We finally went into the pool house, or what they fondly referred to as the Cottage, and it too was perfect. There was only room for one family, which was ideal as it allowed us to set up a little office on the dining room table so we both had a place to work. There was only one caveat: it came with racoons. "They shouldn't bother you," Lydia told us. "But you'll probably hear them walking around in the attic sometimes." We laughed and assured her we were completely fine sharing the space. We had no clue how those racoons would end up playing such an important role in our story!

Chapter 13

We had one final appointment with Blaine's medical oncologist and her staff to go over everything and make sure he was ready to start the chemo. Dr. Baldyga reviewed his lab results and then reminded us of the potential side effects. "Everybody reacts to chemotherapy differently. You may be very nauseated. You may be extra tired. You may develop mouth sores. There are lots of side effects that you may or may not have to deal with. What we know for sure is that you will lose all of your hair and you will have neurological compromise."

We were expecting him to lose his hair, but neurological compromise? What did that mean?

"We know patients undergoing this treatment regimen all have some degree of neurological compromise. They may have problems with their balance. They may have trouble with their speech or their thinking. That can be scary, but we know you will return to normal. We have never had a patient not get back to 100 percent. You just have to ride it out."

I stared at her blankly for a moment, not sure what to do or say. I was prepared for him to have nausea and vomiting and to lose his beautiful hair, but to lose his ability to walk, or to think or communicate clearly? That was a totally different matter. I started to feel a little sick, but I swallowed hard and shoved the feeling down. We were too far into the process to stop now, and besides, she said it wasn't permanent. We could deal with whatever happened as long as it was for a short time. He would ultimately be fine, right?

The day to start killing Lumpy finally arrived. We were ready. The sooner Blaine got started, the sooner this nightmare would be over. We arrived at the main hospital chemotherapy department, the Ambulatory Treatment Center (ATC), a few minutes early, checked in, and sat down to wait.

We waited and waited and then we waited some more. It is impossible to anticipate exactly how long each patient will need. There's no way to know who will get sick or need extra attention, but being the people outside waiting to get started is frustrating . . . and depressing. There are large windows overlooking colorful gardens, but the view outside isn't enough to counterbalance the despair inside. The chemotherapy waiting room is always filled with people going through the worst experience of their lives. Everyone, patients as well as caregivers, looked sick and sad. Several patients were sound asleep with their mouths hanging open and heads lolled off to the side, seemingly beyond caring what anyone thought. I couldn't help staring at them and thinking how awful it must be to have your loved one feel so terrible they would actually fall asleep in a room full of people.

Finally, Blaine's name was called. We followed the nurse through the doors. She took his vital signs and weighed him and then led us to his room. He sat down on the bed and swung his legs around. We gaped at his feet hanging six inches off the end. His 6' 3" frame didn't fit in the bed! I laughed out loud and said, "I thought everything was supposed to be bigger in Texas!"

They eventually got him situated in a room with a bed long enough for him to rest comfortably, and his nurse came in. It was time to get started. I was so scared. I have an unhealthy need to feel in control, to understand exactly why things are happening, and to ensure that everything is as it should be. In addition to earning a degree in sports medicine, I had worked for years as a medical transcriptionist and was knowledgeable about many different medical specialties. I had also worked in medical clinics in third-world countries, and I had grown up with a chronically ill mother who was in and out of the hospital most of my life. I was no stranger to the medical world, but this? This was different. I knew almost nothing, and they were about to infuse actual poison into my favorite person. It should cure him . . . but it just might kill him instead.

Our nurse for the day was David. He confirmed this was Blaine's very first day and began to explain the process to us. "Before we start the chemo, we will give you an infusion of albumin."

"What does the albumin do?" I asked.

David sighed and began again. "Before we start the chemo, we will give you an infusion of albumin. Then we will give you a steroid and then . . ."

"I'm sorry," I interrupted. Why will you give him albumin and a steroid?"

David sighed once more. "Please stop interrupting. Now I have to start over. Before we start the chemo . . ."

My hands began to shake, and blood pulsed through my temples. The person in charge of putting poison into my husband knew so little about it that he only had a memorized speech and wasn't able to answer even one of my questions! I let him continue on while my fear and fury both grew. By the time he was finished, my jaws ached from the effort required to keep from unleashing on him. His eyes darted back and forth between his task and my face. "I don't think your wife likes me very much."

Blaine shot me a look. "Oh, I think she's just a little stressed."

David excused himself to get something and the moment he was out of the room, I hissed, "No way! I'm making them give you someone else. There is *no way* I'm letting him handle this." I was shaking. I am confident I have never been that angry or that scared at any other point in my life.

I was already moving toward the door, but Blaine stopped me. He didn't want to hurt David's feelings. "I'm sure he's totally fine. They wouldn't let him work here if he weren't." I argued, but he was adamant, and it had to be his decision.

David came back in and started the albumin, which we later learned was to give Blaine a little protection against the neurological effects of the chemotherapy. I made him show me the label on each medication before he started it. I'm sure he was annoyed, but I could not have cared less. Blaine was also given two different medications to help ward off the nausea the chemo would cause. One of these, the Decadron, had to be injected very slowly into his IV line or it could possibly cause an "ants in the pants" sensation, according to David. The final pre-med, Emend, came in a normal IV bag and took about thirty minutes to infuse.

Once the Emend was started and I knew it would be a little time before David gave Blaine anything else, I excused myself to find a restroom. There were multiple options inside the chemotherapy suite, but I went out past the waiting area. I locked myself into the stall and finally let the sobs loose that had been threatening all day to overtake me. I've never cried like that in my life. My body shook. I was so scared I could barely breathe. I was a person who needed to have control, and I currently had absolutely none. I had zero understanding of what they were about to put into my husband's body, and the person who was about to do it seemed like he knew nothing. I prayed like I had never prayed before and eventually pulled myself together. I knew I needed to get back in there. David would be coming back soon to put poison into my husband, and even though I really had no way of knowing whether or not he was doing it correctly, I planned to watch every move he made.

Shortly after I arrived back in Blaine's room, David came in with another nurse to start the ifosfamide, the first kind of chemotherapy Blaine was to receive. Both David and the other nurse were donned head to toe with PPE (personal protective equipment), goggles, special gloves, and a special gown covering their clothes. Horror and relief surged through me simultaneously. It was unnerving to realize the substance they were about to infuse inside my husband's body was so dangerous they needed to be protected just to handle it, but realizing David wasn't solely in charge made it a little less terrifying.

The new nurse confirmed Blaine's name and medical record number, and then David read all of the information on the bag of chemo while the other nurse double-checked to make sure everything was right. One of them hooked it to the CVC, and the other one checked to make sure it was done correctly. I soon learned this was standard practice. Every time chemo treatment is initiated, at least two professionals will ensure it is all accurate. Having this knowledge in the beginning would have prevented the bathroom panic attack!

The ifosfamide, along with the mesna to protect Blaine's bladder, took about three hours to infuse. It was all quite uneventful. He didn't burst into flames. He didn't have a heart attack. He didn't start glowing. He watched a movie and napped a little. Some friends had suggested I start a private Facebook group as a way to share information about Blaine's treatment, and while he was asleep, I set that up. It was possibly the best decision I made through this entire ordeal. It allowed me to get information out to hundreds of people with just a few clicks instead of the text after text I had been using to communicate. It also allowed people to remind us they were praying and to send encouragement. It was an absolute lifeline for both of us.

When the ifosfamide was finished, David started some IV Zofran (yet another medicine to help ward off the dreaded nausea) and then some fluid. He and another nurse also came to hook up the pump Blaine would wear for the next twenty-four hours that would infuse another bag of mesna and the second chemotherapy, doxorubicin (mixed with more Zofran). Doxorubicin is known as the "red devil" both for its bright red color as well as the awful side effects it causes. Both medications and a battery-operated pump were placed into a plain black bag Blaine would carry with him everywhere. The doxorubicin and the mesna would be replaced with fresh bags every day.

The nurses gave us detailed descriptions of all the possible things that could go wrong with the pump and how to deal with them. They also had us watch a training film on what to do if somehow any of the chemo should spill and sent us home with a clean-up kit and repeated warnings about how dangerous it was. Thankfully, we never had to use that kit, but it sat in our closet ready to go just in case.

Chapter 14

Every little thing somehow took longer that day than expected. According to our schedule, Blaine was supposed to be in the ATC for five hours, but he was there for a solid eight. Finally, he was finished and ready to go home. He was a little tired but really didn't feel too bad. I was pretty worried about what the evening would bring and quite worried that something would go wrong with his pump, but I pretended not to be. Blaine shouldered the bag, which was pretty heavy with the two full bags of medicine, and walked all the way to the car. I was never able to accurately measure the distance from the ATC to the parking garage, but I'm sure it was close to five miles. Maybe not, but there were certainly days when it felt like it!

We made it back to the Cottage, and Blaine managed to eat a little rice for dinner. We were both exhausted, so we just went to bed as soon as we had finished eating. It was then I first heard the sound. *Whoosh.*

A few seconds later . . . *whoosh.*

It was the pump forcing poison into my husband's body. It was fine while we were up and moving, but once it got quiet, all I could focus on was the *whoosh.* Every time I heard it, a mental image of poison shooting through Blaine's veins flashed across my mind. This went on for about six seconds, and then somehow I heard the *whoosh* and immediately the thought "That's the sound of cancer being killed" came to me. From that moment on, the *whoosh* was soothing, and sometimes I missed it during his off weeks.

Blaine made it through the night without any real problems, other than multiple trips to the bathroom, thanks to the massive amounts of fluid being pumped through him. He wasn't hungry but managed to eat a little breakfast and sat down to check his work email. That's when he had his first big hiccup. Literally, an actual hiccup, followed by another and another. He just kept hiccupping. We did everything we could think of to make them stop, but nothing worked. They weren't regular little hiccups. They were big, shake-his-whole-body hiccups. Every few seconds another one hit him. At first we didn't think too much about them. We assumed they wouldn't last long, but they did. They kept going and going. Blaine said he would much rather have hiccups than the nausea and vomiting we were expecting, but I was worried if they didn't stop soon, they would really start to hurt him.

Today was the beginning of another first for us. In our normal life, Blaine never took medicine. Ever. He had never even been on an antibiotic the entire time I had known him because the few times he was sick, he just toughed it out until he somehow got better. He rarely even agreed to take a Tylenol when he had one of his awful kidney stones. He simply hated taking any sort of medicine.

Now, in addition to the chemotherapy, he was required to take around twenty different prescriptions every day. He had medicines to prevent mouth sores, medicines to prevent nausea, medicines to prevent constipation, medicines to prevent diarrhea, medicines to help his nutritional status. The list went on and on. Some of these had to be taken twice a day, some of them three, some of them four. Some of them couldn't be taken any time near some of the other ones. Some of them had to be taken with food, some on an empty stomach. Some were pills that were easy to swallow, some were gigantic. One had to be crushed into a fine powder. Two had to be swished around his mouth, and one of those had to be swallowed after he swished. Both of those tasted bad. All of them he hated.

Keeping up with his medicine regimen became my full-time job. I was so relieved to find an app for my phone that kept track of the schedule and sent me reminders at the right times. His medications changed constantly, but setting the phone to remind me made it manageable. Trying to keep them scheduled at the right times was hard enough, but making Blaine take them when he felt sick was awful. Frequently they would make him feel bad, but he had to take them so he didn't feel even worse. Being the one responsible for ensuring he got all of it down every day was the worst job I've ever had.

Even with the hiccups, Blaine did finally manage to take all of his medicine for the morning. I packed up everything he would need during the eight hours we might be at the ATC, and we set off.

We arrived at the ATC and sat down to wait . . . and wait. I picked up my phone to scroll through Facebook and was shocked when I realized it was the Fourth of July. I felt so disconnected as I scrolled through everyone's posts showing their fun activities. It didn't seem possible that the world was just continuing on as if everything were normal. Most days I enjoyed seeing what my friends were doing, but it always surprised me to realize normal life was still happening.

At one point, I said something to Blaine, and he didn't answer. I looked over and saw he was sound asleep! I just stared at him. His appearance was changing. He already seemed sickly. It made me feel a little sick myself. It was only the second day! Knowing how desperately I wanted this experience to be over, one of my sisters told me we were "one day closer" every day, and I clung to this, but I knew there were so many days to go.

His name was eventually called. I woke him up, and we headed back to start day two. I was much calmer this time. I was far from comfortable, but knowing what to expect really helped. Being assigned a different nurse also helped. Unfortunately, the hiccups continued. The nurses offered him medicine to make them go away, but he turned them down. He refused to take even one more pill if it was not absolutely necessary. The hiccups went on and on and on. I knew his abdominal muscles must be killing him! Finally, after seven-and-a-half hours, I convinced him to take something to make them stop. The nurse seemed very relieved and hurried out to get them. As soon as she left the room, the hiccups stopped. We couldn't believe the timing! She came back in, and we all had a good laugh. They hooked up fresh bags of the red devil and the mesna and we were finished for the day.

We were about halfway back to the Cottage when the hiccups started up again. I couldn't believe it. They seemed even bigger this time. I felt so bad for Blaine! Of course, we hadn't thought to ask to take the medicine home with us, so we resorted again to every home remedy we had ever heard of. Nothing worked. Every few seconds, his whole body bounced as the hiccup hit him. I finally had the idea of posting about it to his Facebook group and asking for prayer. Because of the timing of the hiccups and the starting and stopping of the doxorubicin, it was evident he was reacting to the chemo, but within an hour of my asking people to pray, the hiccups completely stopped, even though the doxorubicin continued to be pumped into him. I breathed out a huge sigh of relief! We climbed into bed, and Blaine slept peacefully through the night. I was optimistic that the worst was over.

It wasn't. Even though the hiccups stayed away, Blaine started to feel worse and worse as the days went by. We were thankful he never once had any vomiting and didn't even really feel nauseated, but his stomach always just felt sort of unsettled. He had no energy and absolutely no appetite. He was extremely sensitive to any sort of odor and any food that was not room temperature. When he did manage to eat or drink, whatever it was tasted much too salty for him.

As soon as we knew Blaine had cancer, I made plans to ensure he ate lots of healthy foods—no more sugar, no more chemicals, plenty of veggies. All of that went out the window, and I just focused on getting him to eat anything at all that would provide a few calories. The doctors and nurses had also stressed over and over that it was critical he drink lots of water to keep from getting dehydrated. Blaine is not a big drinker of anything, even under the best of circumstances, but now it seemed almost torturous for him to drink. Refrigerated water was too cold, but unrefrigerated water was too warm. Flavored water tasted too strong, but plain water tasted too . . . plain. I ended up mixing refrigerated flavored water with unrefrigerated plain water and pouring a small amount into a little glass. If I gave him too much at a time, he would feel overwhelmed and not drink any, but if I gave him too little, he wouldn't get enough while insisting he didn't need more because he had just finished. It was all such a balancing act, and just when I would feel I had a handle on what he wanted/needed, it would all change.

In addition to the hiccups and sensitivity to taste, another effect of the chemo that we were surprised by is that it made Blaine feel cold. I was determined to do everything I could to make him as comfortable as possible, so we kept the temperature as high as he wanted inside the Cottage. I was so hot! All the time I was hot. Everywhere we went, I was hot (except the hospital; the hospital was always freezing).

As Blaine started to feel worse, I became more and more afraid. As I mentioned earlier, of the two of us, Blaine is always the strong one. He is always the one who remains calm and remembers the important details. That was suddenly totally up to me, and there were *so many* details to keep straight. His life actually depended on my remembering everything, and I was so afraid I would make a mistake. At some point during this time, a Bible verse caught my attention. It says, "Don't panic. I'm with you. There's no need to fear for I'm your God. I'll give you strength. I'll help you. I'll hold you steady, keep a firm grip on you" (Isaiah 41:10 MSG). Soon, I started seeing this verse everywhere—a sign hanging in the hospital, a devotional I read before I went to sleep, random Facebook or Instagram posts. I never mentioned it to anyone, but family and friends started texting it to me out of the blue, saying they had just read it and it made them think of me. That became *my* verse, and I clung to it. As I repeated it over and over to myself, my body relaxed and the jumble in my brain cleared.

Soon, Blaine had finished the fourth day of chemo infusions, and on the fifth day, we went back to the ATC so they could unhook the pump and give him something called Neulasta. This is a medicine that stimulates the bone marrow to make more white blood cells. White blood cells are the body's defense against bacteria that can lead to infection. Chemotherapy works by attacking any fast-growing cells it finds. Unfortunately, white blood cells are fast-growing, so those are attacked also, which means the cancer may be killed, but so may the person's defense against infections.

Neulasta was designed to help with this problem. In order to be the most effective, it needs to be administered twenty-seven hours after the chemo. To alleviate the need for the patient to come back to the hospital again, the Neulasta Onpro was developed. It is a small box with an adhesive back that was placed on Blaine's abdomen. A few seconds later a needle popped out and penetrated his skin to help hold the device in place and in preparation for the medication infusion. He said this didn't hurt, but it startled him every time! That was it. Then we were free to go about our day. We just had to make sure it didn't get wet so it wouldn't come off. This meant he wasn't allowed to sweat, which is hard to prevent in Houston in July, but as he spent almost all of his time inside, where he was freezing, it really wasn't a big deal.

Exactly twenty-seven hours later, it would start beeping and then the medicine would be injected. We knew it took forty-five minutes for all of the medicine to be administered. Blaine just continued doing whatever he was doing and when the time had passed, we checked to make sure it registered as being empty, peeled it off, and threw it in the trash (making sure to put it in something to cover the sharp needle). We had gone into this concerned about Blaine being susceptible to infections, so we were very thankful for this medicine! The drawback is that it can cause severe bone pain. Thankfully, I had read that taking Claritin for a few days (starting the day before the Onpro is applied) helps prevent the pain, and Blaine never had any trouble.

One of the major perks to Blaine's receiving some sort of treatment at the hospital every day is they flushed his CVC lines for me. We were excited to finally reach day six of his cycle because we didn't have to make the trek to the hospital. Unfortunately, now I was solely responsible for making sure his CVC lines were clear and clean.

I was so nervous the first time I flushed them on my own! (Who am I kidding? I was nervous the first twenty-five times!) Thankfully, they had sent us home with step-by-step written instructions. Blaine read each step, and then I followed the directions. Perfect, sterile technique had to be employed. Each lumen had to be wiped with an alcohol wipe for thirty seconds and then allowed to dry for thirty seconds. A small syringe of 0.9 percent sodium chloride then needed to be attached to the lumen and injected up the tube with a push-pause method, ensuring there were no air bubbles.

If the syringe was too tight on the lumen, the fluid would not go in, but if you didn't tighten it enough, the fluid would leak out. Sometimes it would be so hard to inject. Sometimes it went in easily. We had been instructed that Blaine must be taken immediately to the vascular department at the hospital if it ever wouldn't go in at all so they could de-clog it. It was imperative the lines be flushed every single day to keep them free of any bacteria. I was so proud of us when we finished successfully flushing it for the first time! Eventually, this task became just part of our everyday life, and I could pretty much do it in my sleep, but those first few times were scary.

Chapter 15

After he finished the chemo infusions, Blaine felt a little stronger and more like himself every day. We had made it through the first cycle! It certainly wasn't fun, but it hadn't been as bad as we were expecting. He was pretty tired for the first few days after they were over, but soon he was back to working and we settled into a reasonably comfortable routine.

I was so thankful he was feeling better because Kamryn's birthday was rapidly approaching—the only fifteenth birthday she would ever have. The girls had already been by themselves for two weeks. I missed them so much, and the thought of neither parent being there for Kamryn's big day made my heart ache.

Before we left for Texas, some friends gave us their frequent flyer miles. I was overwhelmed by this gift and pretty hesitant to accept it, but they insisted. Dr. Baldyga told us the second week of the upcoming chemotherapy cycles were likely to be the hardest, but she thought it would be okay for me to be gone this first cycle. Blaine's sister, Bobbi, offered to fly down to stay with him, and I used some of the frequent flyer miles to book a round trip back to Springfield.

I was so excited! I was also sad and a little scared. Blaine was feeling better. Honestly, at this point he seemed almost back to normal, but what if something went wrong? I wrote down every little detail that might possibly be important for Bobbi to know. Symptoms necessitating a trip to the ER were taped to the refrigerator where they couldn't be missed. Detailed instructions for all of his medicines and the CVC lines were posted around the Cottage, and I took pictures of all of them to keep on my phone just in case something happened to the multiple copies I had made. I had such mixed feelings about the whole trip. I missed the girls so badly, but thinking about Blaine having a problem while I was away made me sick to my stomach. I was a mess.

Finally, the day arrived. I scheduled an Uber to take me to the airport, threw just a few things into a bag to take with me, and sat down to flush the CVC lines so Bobbi wouldn't have to deal with them on her first day. One line was difficult but finally went through, and I moved on to the next one. I pushed the syringe plunger, but nothing happened. I closed my eyes and took a deep breath, trying to squelch the sense of panic that was quickly settling over me. I tried again. Nothing. Fine beads of sweat broke out on my forehead. This could not be happening. Not now! I tried again and again, but it would not budge. Finally, I looked up and met Blaine's gaze. We both knew we had a big problem.

I called the vascular department, hoping they would tell me it was fine, but of course they confirmed I had to bring him in. If they were able to see him quickly, we would just maybe have enough time to get back before the Uber came to pick me up, assuming the line was easy to fix, but that was a big assumption. We had no clue what would be required. What if he needed surgery to put a brand-new line in?

Although it was not their fault, we knew the vascular department of the hospital struggled even more than the others. In addition to all of their regularly scheduled appointments, they constantly had to deal with people coming in with emergencies, just like we were about to do. If they were backed up, or if Blaine's line had a complicated problem, we would never make it back in time. I said a quick prayer as we rushed to the car.

Thankfully, the traffic between the Cottage and the hospital was not bad, and we found a parking spot easily. We rushed to the vascular department, told them what we needed, and sat down to wait. Of course, the waiting room was full. It didn't look good, but we were shocked to hear his name called after just a few minutes. The nurse led us back to his room, and Blaine sat down on the bed. "So, your line is clogged?" he asked.

I jumped in. "Yes, the white one was tough, but I finally got it. I can't get the orange one at all though."

"Well, sometimes they can be really hard. Let's see if I can get it." He scrubbed the end of the lumen with the antiseptic wipe, let it dry, then attached the syringe of sodium chloride. Then, just as easily as if he were squirting the fluid through the air, he injected it right up the tube. Push, pause, push, pause, push, pause . . . done. I was dumbfounded. I felt like a complete idiot. "Sometimes the blockages disappear by themselves." He gave me a sympathetic smile. "I'm sure that's what happened here." We'll never know for sure if he was right, but I'm choosing to believe it. We raced back to the car and made it to the Cottage with just a few minutes to spare. Nothing like adding a little extra stress to our day!

Once again, I was a little thankful for the rush, as it didn't allow us time to dwell on the fact I was going to be gone for the next several days. Within a few minutes of our arriving back at the Cottage, my Uber arrived. We quickly said goodbye, and I headed for the airport. Bobbi was flying in on the same plane I was flying out on, so Blaine would be alone for a couple of hours, but he seemed fine, and I wasn't worried about him. He never acknowledged this out loud, but I suspect he enjoyed having some time to himself.

Chapter 16

In addition to all my worries about my not being there to care for Blaine, there was another major concern: COVID. The week I was flying home, Springfield, Missouri, had the highest percentage of COVID cases in the country. We had been so careful not to be exposed, but now I was about to get on a plane, where I would be surrounded by potentially infectious people. If I got COVID and exposed Blaine, it would cause a major delay in his treatment, but of course the bigger worry was if he were to catch it from me. Even with the Neulasta, we knew his ability to fight off an infection was weakened. Would he survive a case of COVID? We had no way of knowing, and I was terrified to find out. The girls had been quarantining as best as possible, and we had plans in place to continue to be very cautious while I was home, but there was nothing I could do about the airplane.

I double-masked before I went into the airport and sat down to wait as far away from the other passengers as possible. The plane arrived, and I chatted with Bobbi for a few minutes before it was time to board. As I feared, the flight was completely full. I was seated in the very last row by the window. I was feeling a little claustrophobic and a lot irritated, but then I realized I was really only being directly exposed to the person sitting right next to me. No one was behind to breathe on me and there was not anyone on my other side. If I had to be on a packed plane, I was probably in the safest seat!

The flight was uneventful, and I rushed out to meet the girls. Kaia pulled up, and an instant later the four of us were gripped in a giant hug right on the sidewalk. I couldn't hold back my smile as I squeezed them with all my strength. I had missed them so much! The two weeks I had been away felt like two years. Thankfully, they had brought me dinner, and I inhaled it while Kaia drove home, and everyone tried to talk at once. We had communicated every day while I was gone, but there was still so much to say! When we arrived home, the dogs went berserk. They were so funny! Between the dogs and the girls, I felt very loved and knew I had been missed. Crawling into my own bed that night was glorious.

The next morning was not so glorious. All I could think about was the fact that if Blaine died, it would just be the girls and me in the house, exactly like it was now. I spent most of the day crying and trying to hide it, but the girls could tell. In my head, I knew Blaine had a decent prognosis, but I also knew we couldn't count on things turning out the way we were hoping. It was an awful day. I was so happy to be home with Kaia, Kaci, and Kamryn, but I felt so guilty for leaving Blaine, and I could not stop wondering if this wasn't a picture of what my future would be like.

My guilt was about to get worse. I called Blaine first thing that morning to see how he was doing. He didn't answer, but my phone buzzed a moment later. My breath caught in my chest as I read his text. "I'm sorry I couldn't answer. My throat, mouth, and tongue feel like they're on fire."

I never should have left him! What was I thinking? I was a horrible wife. I had been gone less than a day, and now the side effect I feared the most was happening. Other than that, he said he felt okay. He planned to drink lots of lukewarm tea and do some work.

A few hours later, Bobbi called to break the news I had been dreading. Blaine was running a fever! Any sort of fever when one is receiving chemotherapy is considered an emergency. We had been instructed to take Blaine's temperature at least four times every day and alert them about any elevations. If it hit 100.1, he had to immediately be taken to the closest emergency room. I was almost 700 miles away, and now he had a fever! He and Bobbi kept me updated throughout the day. His temperature would inch up and then go back down a little, then inch up a little more, but there was no doubt it was definitely climbing. She spoke with the on-call oncologist several times, and they were going back and forth as to whether Blaine needed to come in. Of course, he did not want to go.

Finally, Blaine noticed his finger was a little swollen and had a tiny cut. Bobbi called the doctor who confirmed Blaine's defenses were probably so low this little break in the skin was causing him to run the fever. He instructed them to put some regular antibiotic ointment on it and to watch it closely. That did the trick. The next day his fever was gone, and his finger looked much better. A day later, his sore throat, mouth, and tongue were much better too. Hopefully the worst was over! I felt so bad I hadn't been there to take care of him, but he and Bobbi had handled it just fine. I needed to relax and enjoy my time with the girls.

The next day was Kamryn's birthday. It didn't seem possible that the baby of our family was fifteen years old! We Face-Timed with Blaine while she opened her presents, and that evening her friend's mom threw a little party for her and a few of her friends. I was so thankful for this! I desperately needed to know Kamryn would have fun memories from her big day, but I just did not have it in me to put something together. The moms were invited too, and it was so good for me to visit with people and do something normal for a few hours, even if I had to keep my distance to make sure I didn't pick up any germs.

The next morning, I took Kamryn for her driver's permit test. As expected, she passed with flying colors. I flashed her my biggest smile, but inside a million worries competed for my attention. There was no way to know how the next year would look for us. Would Blaine be up to teaching her to drive? He had taught the other two girls. That was his job. I teach academic subjects; he teaches them to drive. That's the deal. I wanted no part of that, but I had no idea how she was going to learn.[8]

A few days later, I was having a lovely time visiting with my friend, Traci, at our favorite coffee shop when my phone buzzed and I looked down to see a simple, five-word text from Blaine: "My hair is falling out." Nothing ruins a good cup of coffee like the jolting reminder that your husband is sick and is indeed going to lose his beautiful hair. It should not have been a surprise, but so much time had passed, I had secretly started to believe that maybe, just maybe, it wouldn't happen to him, that his hair was indeed so wonderful, it was strong enough to resist chemotherapy. No such luck. I let out a huge sigh.

"What's wrong?" Traci asked. I showed her the text, and she let out her own sigh. Traci had walked through this with her husband a few years earlier. She knew what this meant. She understood it represented so much more than just hair. I texted back something encouraging and moved on with my day. I was scheduled to fly back in a few days, and there was a lot to be done. There was no time to mourn the hair.

My time at home was passing quickly. I did all the home maintenance things that needed to be done. I got the bills caught up and restocked the groceries so the girls would have plenty to eat the next two weeks until we were home. I also tried to spend as much time with Kaia as possible. I could not believe I had waited the entire school year for her to come home and then missed out on most of her time. I was going to have to leave again, then come back just in time to take her back to school. Who knew how long it would be before we saw her again after that? She was building her own life away from us. I had a sinking feeling this would be her last summer at home, and I had missed it! It wasn't fair. Every time I thought about it, I wanted to punch something and bawl my eyes out at the same time. There was no way to fix it, so I just tried to make the most of the time we had together.

After cramming as much into the day as possible, I fell into bed completely worn out, and then lay there awake for hours, just like I did almost every night. For weeks I had been utterly exhausted, but I could not sleep.

I simply could not make my brain quiet down. I wasn't even necessarily worried; it was just a matter of there being so many things to keep track of. Did I remember all of Blaine's pills? Were the girls eating healthy food? Should I make Blaine get exercise or let him sleep? Does Kaci have a ride to work? Is the nurse doing the chemo right? Are the girls making good choices? A friend told me about the colonoscopy she had earlier in the week. She said it was the best sleep she's ever had, and I wondered if maybe I shouldn't get one—just so I could get in a decent nap!

Earlier that day I had asked Blaine if I should post to his Facebook group about his hair falling out. He said I should, that he wanted to be real through this. I decided if he could be real, then I should be also, and the next day I posted about my sleeping issue. Many people promised to pray, and there is no doubt their prayers helped, but a few told me privately they sometimes used Benadryl to help them sleep. I decided to try it. I have always been concerned about developing an addiction, and I was afraid taking something to help me sleep would be a slippery slope, but I was desperate, so I tried it anyway. It's not an exaggeration to say it may have saved me. I was very careful not to take one too many nights in a row, but it was extremely helpful when I did.

My week at home flew by and seemed to take forever all at the same time. Wanting desperately to be in two different places simultaneously sometimes made me wonder if I was going crazy. Good or bad, the day of my flight back to Texas finally arrived. We had taken COVID precautions while I was home, but there was once again nothing I could do about the germs I would be exposed to on the flight back. I said goodbye to the girls, double masked myself, and headed back into the airport. I found my gate and groaned as I saw the crowd of people waiting for my flight. I sat as far away from everyone as possible and waited for the time to board. I was sad to be leaving the girls but not horribly. I knew we would be back in less than two weeks. We had survived the first part of this ordeal. The second part would be fine.

It was finally time to board. My row was empty, and I settled in, savoring the moment of not being crowded between strangers but knowing it wouldn't last long. My head jerked up in surprise as I heard the flight attendant close the door. I was still alone! I glanced around the plane in awe as I saw every other row was full except the ones directly behind, in front of, and across from mine. Those were completely empty. God had provided a ring of safety for me. I sat back in my seat and relaxed, reminded once more that God was taking care of us!

When the plane landed, I was able to visit with Bobbi for a few minutes before she boarded to fly back to Springfield, and then I headed out to meet my Uber. I texted Blaine to let him know I was on my way. He texted back a few minutes later, "Consider yourself warned. After Bobbi left, I shaved my beard. It was falling out in big clumps, and I decided to just get it over with."

I leaned back against the seat. My mind raced with a million thoughts at once. I had never seen him without facial hair, and I couldn't even picture how he was going to look. I hated that it was falling out, and I hated that he had to deal with it alone, but I was also relieved I didn't have to watch. "Well, okay!" I texted back. "Can't wait to see you!"

The Uber pulled up to the house, and my new clean-faced husband came out to meet me. He looked completely different! It was shocking, and I was glad he had warned me. I jumped out of the Uber and ran to hug him. Beard or no beard, it was so good to see him! He was clearly self-conscious, but I assured him he looked great. I think losing his beard might have been the hardest part of the whole cancer experience for him.

Chapter 17

By the next day, it was evident the hair on Blaine's head was going too. His hairline just kept moving further and further back. He seemed to age twenty years every few hours. Finally, he got tired of watching it and announced it was time. I had brought his electric razor from home. We spread a sheet out on the floor, and I shaved off his beautiful hair. It was harder than I had expected, not emotionally harder—somehow I managed not to really think about it—but it was physically hard to get it all off. Whereas the hair on the front of his head fell out if you looked at it funny, the hair on the back was determined to stay. We never could get his scalp to be perfectly smooth like I had envisioned, but we got as much hair off as possible. He definitely looked different, definitely like a cancer patient, but he was still cute!

The next morning was prep time for cycle two. Blaine had labs and a chest X-ray to make sure the CVC was still in place and ready to receive the chemo, and he met with Dr. Baldyga and her staff to go over the plan. The plan was the same. They were pleased with how the first cycle went, and while we couldn't say we were *pleased*, it hadn't been as bad as we were expecting. We were anxious for the next cycle to get started so it could be done. At the end, he would be one-third of the way finished, and we would be able to go home for a couple weeks! "One day closer. One day closer," I repeated over and over to myself.

Day one of cycle two was so much better for me. Knowing what to expect makes such a difference! We walked into the chemotherapy waiting room different people than we were the last time. We weren't the terrified newbies. We belonged here. These were our people, even though we didn't know any of them.

There's something special about cancer patients and the people who love them. I've often heard the phrase, "Be kind. Everyone is fighting a battle you know nothing about." In this waiting area, in this hospital, everyone was fighting a battle, and we knew exactly what it was. Amazingly, everyone was kind. It's a different world in so many ways, and one of them is definitely how kind the people are. Although most people didn't really talk much, someone would always hold an elevator, pick something up if you dropped it, or offer directions if you looked lost. No one ever tried to cut in line, and I only heard someone raise their voice once. Considering how much stress we were all under, this amazed me.

At least once every day, some random person would smile at me, and I was always surprised how much this tiny gesture helped my mood. I decided that was something easy I could do to help others, so I made it my personal mission to smile at people as I passed them. I hoped that would bring them at least a moment of peace, but I suspect it may have actually helped me even more.

Day one went smoothly, and soon we were back at the Cottage. Blaine managed to eat a little and went to bed. Just as I started to doze off, the bed shook. The hiccups were back, and they were huge. Every few seconds the whole bed bounced! This time I didn't wait as long to post on Facebook and ask people to pray. Before long, they stopped and he was able to get some sleep. They would come and go over the next few days, but thankfully they never lasted as long as they did that first time. He insisted he would rather have hiccups than nausea, but I know they must have been painful.

The next day while Blaine was getting his chemo, I walked over to the pharmacy to pick up some of his medications. This was always a stressful trip for me. My whole life I had worried about money. Now, we were hemorrhaging money. I tried so hard not to think about it, but the worry constantly lingered in the back of my mind. As always, there was a line, but finally it was my turn. I gave the tech Blaine's medical record number, which I had thankfully memorized, and he brought me the big bag of medicine. "Here you go. Have a nice day."

"How much do I owe you?"

"Nothing. It looks like it's covered."

I couldn't believe it! I was walking out with at least $100 worth of medicine, and I hadn't been charged for any of it! I assumed it was a glitch and I ultimately was going to be billed, but for the moment, it made my day. I walked back to Blaine's room and told him, and it made his day too.

Over the next few hours, though, the realization of why we hadn't been charged dawned on me. We had reached our out-of-pocket maximum for our insurance. Suddenly, my day was no longer made. The knowledge that we now had a $16,000 medical bill settled over me like a heavy, wet blanket. Of course, I knew it was going to happen, but . . . that was so much money! Eventually, I was able to shove the worry to the back of my mind. It didn't matter. It was just money. We would keep paying on it, and eventually it would be paid off. Ultimately, this was a good thing. I didn't worry in the slightest if Blaine needed some additional freakishly expensive test or if the girls needed something. All of our medical expenses for the rest of the year were totally covered.

The rest of the treatment time went smoothly, and soon we were on our way out of the department. Blaine had his red devil bag, and we were walking back to the parking garage. Suddenly he stopped and then just almost fell over. "What are you doing?" I asked, a little rougher than I intended because he scared me.

"I had to burp."

"And that made you fall over?"

"You know I've never been good at multitasking."

I just stared at him. Before I knew what was happening, my stomach started to shake. I tried as hard as I could to choke it down, but it was impossible to control. First a tiny snort escaped, then a giggle, and a second later I was doubled over, laughing uncontrollably. Blaine stared at me for a split-second, and then he was laughing too. We were standing in the middle of a busy hallway in one of the saddest places on earth laughing like we didn't have a care in the world. We may have both been a little slap-happy, but it just struck me as the funniest thing ever. He regained his balance, managed not to burp anymore, and we made our way to the car without incident. It really wasn't funny. It was a sign of the neurological compromise we had been worried about, and we both knew it, but it is still one of my favorite memories of the whole ordeal.

The next two days passed easily, and just like that, the infusion part of cycle two was over. They unhooked his pump, put on the Neulasta, and sent us home. They had warned us days four through seven would likely be the time when he felt the worst, and they were not wrong. He didn't get the vomiting we were so afraid of, and the dreaded hiccups were fairly mild, but he just felt icky and really, really tired, so he spent the vast majority of his time in bed. I worked some, kept on top of his medicine regimen, and watched some TV. The whole day, I just kept feeling warmer and warmer. Blaine was already miserable, so I knew I couldn't make the air cooler, but I felt as if I were living in an oven.

I finally decided it was time to go to bed. I was hoping Blaine would be sound asleep and wouldn't notice if I turned the air down just a bit. I walked into our bedroom and was surprised to see he had thrown the covers off. That was strange. He was always freezing. I went to turn down the AC and noticed the thermostat said it was ninety degrees in the house. No wonder I was so hot! The air was blowing. What in the world was going on? I reached up to the vent and felt hot air on my hand. I couldn't believe the luck. The whole reason we were in the Cottage was because the air conditioning wasn't working in the other house. Now this one was broken?

I wasn't sure what to do. I was determined not to be any trouble for Lydia or Mercy House Ministries. I didn't want to call and say we needed them to get it fixed, but could we really survive in Houston with no air conditioning? It was 10:30 at night, and it was still so hot outside I couldn't decide if opening the windows would help cool the house down or just make it worse. I finally decided to keep the windows closed and hoped turning off the lights would help enough to let me sleep. I had actually just started to doze off when I remembered Blaine had the Neulasta box on. The directions specifically stated he could not sweat and there was no way he was not sweating! I decided there was nothing I could do about it besides pray, so I posted to the Facebook group, said a quick prayer myself, and went to sleep.

First thing the next morning, I gave in and called Lydia. She assured me she would get someone right out. She must have some pull because the repairmen were at the house within the hour. They looked all around and could not find anything wrong. Finally, they decided they needed to go into the attic to look at the equipment there. The only access to the attic was through the bedroom where Blaine was trying to rest, but it couldn't be helped.

As soon as they got up there, they saw the problem. The lid to a safety valve had been taken off and was on the other side of the attic. The racoons must have been playing with it. Until then, they had never bothered us. We loved listening to them running around up there, but now we had a problem. The repairman put the lid back on the valve, and within seconds, it began blowing cold air again.

There was no way to know that the racoons wouldn't just take it off again, or do something worse, so Lydia decided it was time for them to go. She called the Texas Parks and Wildlife Department and they agreed to come out as soon as possible. Of course, they were going to have to go through the bedroom to get to the attic. Blaine said he didn't care. I was sure they would take just a few minutes to capture them in some non-stressful way and take them off to spend the remainder of their days living it up in the woods somewhere. Then Blaine would be free to rest all he needed, and we wouldn't have to worry about what damage they might be doing.

That's not exactly the way it played out.

Chapter 18

Poop. That's how it played out. With poop. That evening, Mike from the Texas Parks and Wildlife Department came to take care of the racoons. He introduced himself to poor Blaine, who was still in the bed, and apologized for having to disturb him. He choked up while he told us his wife had been a patient at MDA for a brain tumor and assured us Blaine was in the best possible hands. Then he said, "It won't take me long. I'll just put this poop up there real fast, and then I'll be out of your hair."

Surely I must have misheard him. "I'm sorry. Did you say 'poop'?"

"Oh yes, that's the best way to get rid of racoon families. We put male racoon poop where they're staying. The momma thinks there's a male around who might hurt her babies, so she moves them somewhere she thinks is safer. I'm sure they'll leave tonight."

He went up to spread the poop all around the attic, assured us that would take care of the problem, then went home to his now-healthy wife. Unfortunately, I was now alone with my very sick, very sensitive-to-smells-husband in a house with buckets of actual raccoon poop. This was certainly not a problem I had anticipated! Now we had air conditioning, but I propped all the doors open to get the smell out. Then I posted an update on the Facebook group asking them to pray for protection from raccoon poop. My life was so weird.

Surprisingly it wasn't as bad as I had expected, and by the time I went to bed, even Blaine could barely smell it, so we shut all the doors and went to sleep. The smell was completely gone the next morning. We both agreed we would miss hearing the raccoons, but we were glad we didn't have to worry about their doing any more damage.

The next morning, I dropped Blaine off for his last set of labs before we headed home. Hospital parking is expensive, so whenever possible, Blaine went in by himself and I found somewhere else to wait. Today, I drove to McDonald's, enjoyed a coffee under the palm trees, and then went back to pick him up. By this point, I had gotten quite comfortable with the layout of the hospital and the roads surrounding it and made the drive without even thinking. I was so excited to be going home! I belted out a song with the radio as I scanned the pickup area looking for Blaine. As always, there were several very old, very sick-looking patients sitting there waiting. Suddenly, I slammed on my brakes. One of those very old, very sick-looking people was my husband! I didn't recognize him and had almost driven right by.

I felt terrible but covered well, and I don't think he ever had any idea. My good mood vanished. I was taken aback by how bad he looked and couldn't believe I hadn't noticed before. Maybe it just took being away from him for a bit to see with fresh eyes. It hit me then how shocked the girls were going to be, and it broke my heart to know they were going to have that experience. I really didn't want this to be part of their lives. I knew at this point in the cycle, he should start feeling a little better every day. Hopefully by the time we got home tomorrow night, he wouldn't look quite so awful. I plastered a smile on my face, acted like everything was just fine, and drove us back to the Cottage to pack.

We were ready to head home first thing in the morning. I had just finished packing the last of our stuff when the phone rang, and I looked down to see Dr. Baldyga's nurse was calling.

"Hi, Veronica!" I answered brightly. I always enjoyed talking with her, and I assumed she was calling to wish us well on our trip home.

"Hi, Mrs. Parker." She got right to the point. "I have some bad news. Blaine's labs aren't good. They show he is very dehydrated, and it's affecting his kidney function. You need to get him to the ER for fluids and potassium as soon as possible."

We left immediately. MD Anderson has its own emergency department. It was comforting to know they had all his records and knew exactly what treatment would be needed to most effectively deal with the side effects of his particular chemotherapy regimen. I had driven past the ER almost every day and made a point to notice how to get there, but I had really hoped he would never need to go.

We parked and walked in to discover the waiting room was completely packed! The hospital took great pains to socially distance the patients, but here there simply was no choice but to have everyone crowded in together. I had mistakenly believed since the ER was only for MDA patients, it would never be crowded. I did learn later that the weekdays are typically much busier than Saturdays and Sundays, the exact opposite of what I would have expected, because most people had labs done during the week and then got sent to the ER, exactly like we were.

Finally, a couple of seats opened up, and we sat down to wait for Blaine's turn. Nine hours later, after bags of IV fluid and potassium, we were heading back to the Cottage. I was shocked to discover there was still traffic in Houston at 1:30 in the morning, but it was much better than normal.

We pulled in the driveway and tried to sneak back to the Cottage as quietly as possible, hoping not to disturb Lydia and her husband, and went right to bed. We were supposed to be leaving for home in five hours. Obviously, that was not going to happen, and I was heartbroken and filled with guilt that I was heartbroken.

Spending nine hours in the ER of a cancer hospital is not an experience I would ever wish on anyone. As sick as Blaine was, he was not nearly as sick as most of the other patients. The vast majority did not get to leave the hospital. Some of them died that night. I was curled up next to my, all things considered, completely fine husband in my very comfortable home-away-from-home feeling sorry for myself. I knew all of that. I knew in the grand scheme of things, my situation wasn't anywhere close to being as sad as it could be, but I was still so, so sad. I missed the girls so much! I missed my friends and my dogs and my peaceful little town with its abundance of cows and reasonable number of cars.

The next morning, I called the girls to let them know we weren't going to make it home that day. I had kept them updated on our trip to the ER, so they weren't surprised, but we now had a major problem. Kaia had an appointment with her surgeon, six hours away, that she could not miss, and she had no way to get there. Finally, it was decided that her boyfriend, Hunter, would drive down to get her.

I was so thankful for this and so demoralized by this all at the same time. I was happy to know she had people in her life who would drop what they were doing and spend two days making sure she got where she needed to be, but I had desperately been looking forward to that time with her. Maybe even more than that, it was a sign that we really weren't needed as much as I liked to think we were. Our children's lives were continuing on just fine even though we were barely a part of them. Every parent has to adjust to their children becoming adults, but most of them get to ease into it slowly. For us, it had happened pretty much overnight, and one of them was barely fifteen.

During our entire ordeal, this day was one of the hardest for me. A friend called, and while I always made a great effort to give the impression I was okay, she knew I wasn't. She also knew I couldn't let Blaine know how devastated I was and told me I needed to make an excuse to go to the store and give myself some time just to cry. I still had the idea that crying was pointless, and honestly, I was a little bit afraid if I started I might never stop, but I did it anyway, and it did help. Maybe it wasn't so pointless after all.

Chapter 19

The sun rose the next morning, and so did we. It's amazing what a good night's sleep will do. I was still so disappointed we weren't able to go home but had accepted it. There was no other choice. We would do what we needed to do, and each day would bring us one day closer to getting back to our real life.

Kaia's stuff was loaded into Hunter's car, and they drove to Iowa so she could start her second year of college. Kaci sent me a picture of her waving goodbye, and while I was still sad to be missing this time with her, I was also proud. Kaia actually had been born in China, and the name given to her from the orphanage where she lived, HuaPing, means "beautiful and resilient." We had thought that was such a perfect name for her, but it turned out it was going to apply to her sisters as well. All of them were beautiful and resilient, and while I missed them like crazy, I woke up that morning thankful God had made them so strong.

Blaine also woke up that morning feeling much better! We watched a church service online, and then he spent the afternoon catching up on work and blaring spaghetti western music and singing along. I stared at him in awe, amazed at how quickly he had bounced back! It was a good day, and things were definitely looking up. Tomorrow he would have labs, and surely the day after that we would finally head home.

When I took him in for labs the next day, he was feeling fine, almost totally normal. I picked him up when he was finished, and we went back to the Cottage to work. We had kept all of our things packed and were ready to leave first thing in the morning. All we had to do was wait for the call from Dr. Baldyga's office confirming Blaine's blood work looked good.

Finally, the phone rang. "Hello Mrs. Parker. We have Blaine's lab results. We have good news and bad news." My heart sank a little as I braced myself for the bad part of her news. "Blaine's kidney function is looking much better. Unfortunately, his phosphorus and potassium levels have fallen even further."

In my head, I thought, "So? Increase his supplements. Big deal. We're going home. Nothing can stop us."

She went on, "Unfortunately, that's not the bad news. Blaine's white count is 0.5. A normal white count is between 4 and 11. He has almost no defense against infection. I understand you're planning on driving to southern Missouri tomorrow?"

"Yes," I said with a sinking feeling.

"You need to consider that very carefully. It is, of course, your choice, but if you go, you must take his temperature every two hours, and if he registers any sort of fever at all, you must take him immediately to the closest emergency room."

I pictured the drive in my mind. Without stops, it would take us close to eleven hours to get home, and we would drive for hours through the countryside, where there would be no hospital anywhere close. Frankly, once we left Houston, there was only one city that would have an ER I might feel comfortable taking him to, and of course, there was COVID.

"And of course, he must not, under any circumstances, be exposed to COVID. He simply has zero resources to fight any virus, and COVID will be extremely, extremely dangerous for him. My understanding is that COVID is particularly prevalent in southern Missouri right now. Is that right?"

"Yes."

Silence.

More silence.

Finally, I thanked her for calling and assured her we would not leave town anytime soon. As desperately as I wanted to go home, I absolutely would not risk Blaine's life for it. I hung up the phone and went to unpack our things.

Chapter 20

The next morning, I had a long, honest talk with Dr. Baldyga. She confirmed my fear that most likely Blaine's white count would now fall after every single cycle of chemo. It should rebound by the third week, and he would likely feel pretty good, but if we waited until the third week to go home, we would only have a couple of days there before we needed to return to Houston. If we were going to go home, we absolutely must leave immediately after the infusion was completed in order to get there before his white count fell. Unfortunately, he always felt pretty miserable the first couple of days after he received the chemo, and a long trip would be difficult; not to mention that would put him in the COVID capital of the country during the week he had no defense. It just didn't make sense.

He still had three-and-a-half more months of chemotherapy immediately followed by five weeks of radiation. We were going to have to stay in Houston for five more months —and that was if there were no delays in the treatment schedule, which we knew was a pretty big *if*. I just couldn't wrap my head around this. What had happened to our lives? When they initially told us we needed to stay in Houston for a week for the first tests, I thought that was such a big deal. We were now going to have to stay for six months. Six months! How were Kaci and Kamryn supposed to live by themselves for six months? Blaine's company had approved his being gone for one month, not half a year! How was that going to work?

There was no choice. We had to accept it and move on. I broke the news to Lydia, and she assured me she was fine with us living in her backyard for five more months, or as long as we needed. I breathed out a huge sigh of relief! Mercy House Ministries is only able to provide housing for patients for a maximum of three months, but since the Cottage was Lydia's personal property, she could make her own rules. I had mistakenly believed God had arranged the Cottage just so we would have a pleasant place to stay for the month we were there, and I'm sure that was part of it, but He knew what was coming, and he had provided a way through even before we knew there was a need.

I called Kaci and Kamryn to let them know we weren't going to be able to come home that week and updated Kaia on what was going on. They asked when we would be home, and I had no answer for them. I'm sure this was extremely unsettling. Their mother always had a plan. Now I simply had to tell them I had no clue what was going to happen.

As if our disappointment weren't enough, as expected, Dr. Baldyga increased the supplements to ensure Blaine had enough phosphorus and potassium in his system, and that made him feel really sick. To help with this, she put him on more medicine. Now he was taking medicine to protect him from the medicine he was taking to protect him from the medicine. For a man who very rarely ever took a Tylenol in his normal life, this was getting completely out of hand, but there was nothing we could do about it.

As disappointed as I was not to be on my way home, it turned out to be good we had stayed. As always, I took Blaine's temperature several times a day. It had always stayed right around normal. That afternoon, however, it was just a little higher. I didn't think too much about it but took it again a few hours later. It was a little bit higher than the time before. At this point, I started to worry and was thankful we weren't somewhere in the middle of nowhere on our way home, but when I took it again an hour later, it was back to normal. Good! I had worried for nothing.

An hour later it was higher again. It wasn't to the 100.1 threshold we knew mandated an ER trip, but it was starting to get closer. The weird thing was that sometimes when I would take it, it would be lower, but then the next time it would be higher. It was maddening, and I started to question the reliability of our digital thermometer. At some point that evening, Lydia stopped by, and I mentioned what was happening. She came back a few minutes later with an old-fashioned mercury thermometer. I was a tiny bit concerned I would have trouble reading it, but when I took it out of his mouth, it was as clear as could be: 101.8.

101.8! My heart started racing, but I forced myself to act perfectly calm. "Your temperature is 101.8. We need to go to the ER." I expected him to argue, but he didn't hesitate. We got there in record time, and I pulled up to the door to drop him off. His oncology team had stressed repeatedly that I must always know what day of his cycle he was on, and I was prepared. "When you walk in, tell them you are on day eleven, your white count is 0.5, and you have a fever of 101.8." Blaine hates being told what to do, and he never wants to make a big deal about any medical issue, but he just said, "Okay," and walked in. I found a parking spot quickly, and by the time I got inside, they already had him in a room and were just finishing taking his temperature. It was 99.3.

I felt like crying. What in the world? I considered it a small miracle that Blaine had agreed to go to the ER. If I had made him go for no reason, it was going to be really difficult to get him to go again if he needed to. "I promise it was 101.8. I even checked it on a regular mercury thermometer," I told the doctor.

"I am sure that it was," the doctor replied. "Neutropenic fevers, meaning fevers that the body produces in response to a super low white count, frequently rise and fall. I'm not surprised at all that it's lower now. It will probably go back up in a little while."

"So I was right to bring him in?"

"Absolutely! With his white count this low, even this tiny elevation means he needs antibiotics. His body has no ability to fight anything on its own. We don't mess around with that."

I felt so much better! I was scared he was sick, but at least I knew I had made the right decision. They ran lots of tests, but didn't find any particular infection, which they said is pretty common. They did discover his white count had now fallen to 0.3, and his platelets were just barely above the level mandating a transfusion. They gave him two different kinds of IV antibiotics and sent him home with a prescription for a third. Surely that would kill any germs!

We were so focused on Blaine's health, I wasn't paying attention to the calendar. The next morning I turned on my computer to get a little work done and gasped when the date flashed across the screen. It was my favorite day of the year: Blaine's birthday! He is four months younger than I am. Those are the longest four months of the year because he loves to tease me about being older. I wished we could do something fun to celebrate, but instead we had to go back to the hospital so they could check his labs again. He felt so awful! I hated making him get up and leave the house. We stopped at a stoplight, and I glanced over at him and my heart just broke. He looked so miserable. Honestly, he looked like he was dying, and for the first time, I prayed that if he was going to die, God would just take him quickly. It was an awful, awful moment, but I loved him so much, and as much as the thought of living without him hurt, the thought of him having to feel like this for very long hurt even more.

He went in and had his blood drawn, and again I was so very thankful for the CVC line so he didn't have to get stuck with a needle. We drove back to the Cottage, and he went straight to bed while I obsessively waited for his results to be posted. It didn't take long. Good news: his white count was up to 1.8, still a far cry from 4, but most definitely better than yesterday. Unfortunately his platelets had fallen further. No wonder he felt so bad! I waited for them to call to tell me to bring him back in for a transfusion, but the call never came, and weirdly enough, Blaine started to feel better. His energy didn't last long, but he had a few hours when he felt pretty decent. His aunt had arranged for a birthday cake and a nice dinner to be delivered, and Lydia brought us both presents. It was most definitely not the birthday I was hoping for, but it turned out much better than I had expected at the beginning of the day.

Chapter 21

As confident as Mike from the Texas Parks and Wildlife Department had been that the male racoon poop would inspire our little family to move on, he was wrong. We heard them all the time running around in the attic. One morning, after they had been particularly noisy through the night, I opened the door, planning to climb up and see if they had done any damage. Before I could pull the steps down, a little masked baby face poked out. He was so cute! I loved hearing them running around, and I really didn't want them to go. However, I also loved air conditioning, so I knew having them live with us was a problem.

When it became obvious they were not afraid of male racoons, Lydia called Mike to let him know he needed to try something else. She told me he was nice but clearly distracted. He informed her he would come back out as soon as he could, but right now their department was dealing with a bigger problem: killer bees. I had read about killer bees in Texas a few months earlier, but I assumed it was just a joke. It wasn't. There were actual killer bees in Houston, and now they were near our house. Clearly that trumped our little racoon problem, but he would get back to us when he could. Lydia told him not to worry, that we would definitely rather deal with raccoons than bees and to please take care of them first!

After a few days, the wildlife department had successfully gotten rid of the killer bees, and Mike came back to deal with us. He decided he would wait for the raccoons to leave for their evening foraging and then simply board up the hole where they were accessing the attic. He climbed up on our roof and mounted a camera so he could watch for them. Once everything was up and running, he went back to his truck to wait.

It felt a little weird knowing someone was sitting in the driveway watching our house, but so many things now felt weird in our lives that we didn't think much about it. At some point in the night, I heard him on the roof hammering a cover over their access hole. I was a little sad to think about them coming back and not being able to get into their home but thankful we no longer had to worry about them doing any damage.

A little while later we awoke to a ruckus. *BANG! BANG, BANG, BANG, BANG, BANG!* The raccoons were still up there. Mike had mistakenly locked them in instead of out, and they were furious! *BANG, BANG, BANG, BANG!* They were going completely crazy! For hours we listened while they tore the place to pieces. The door with the stairs in our bedroom bounced up and down as they tried everything to get out, even attempting to go through our room. *BANG, BANG, BANG!* It was a very long night. I could imagine how scared they must be, knowing they were trapped. The little lid to the air conditioner valve didn't stand a chance. After several hours of this, they did finally settle down and miraculously never messed with the AC. First thing in the morning, Lydia called Mike, and he came and removed the barricade. He would have to come up with another plan.

If we were not going to be able to go home for the next few months, among the million little problems, there was one giant problem: Kamryn's school. As we were a homeschooling family, I was in charge of every aspect of Kamryn's education, and that was a responsibility we took very seriously. All of her curriculum for the upcoming year, her first year of high school, had been purchased the previous spring, so, thankfully, that was ready to go, but how was she supposed to do a full semester of school without a teacher?

Many of her friends had done school virtually when everything was closed for COVID. That's what we would have to do. It certainly wasn't ideal, but nothing about this situation was ideal. That meant I would need books and schedules with me, and she would need access to everything at home. Blaine continued to feel a little bit better every day, and the doctor confirmed his white count should be high enough by the beginning of week three for him to safely be around another person. His friend, Chris, graciously offered to come stay with him so I could fly home to reorganize the school plan and get the materials I needed to have with me.

I was only going to be home for a few days, and there was so much to do! My first day home, once again I was struck with the sense that if Blaine died, this was what our house would feel like. I hated that so much and really struggled to be productive, but I simply did not have time to waste.

In normal years, I spend most of the summer preparing everything for the upcoming school year. I put together lesson plans for each week and schedules for the whole year so we stay on track to complete everything on time. I make all the copies, and I organize everything so it's easy to find. This year I only had three days, and I needed to structure things so I could teach from a distance, not really having any idea what my day-to-day life was going to look like.

I knew things had to be arranged so that if necessary, Kamryn could do as much as possible on her own. I switched a few subjects to more student-directed curriculums, and I hired a teacher for algebra. I made copies of anything I thought I might possibly need and organized everything so Kamryn would know exactly where it was. I wanted so desperately to keep her on schedule and not let this cancer thing change her life any more than absolutely necessary. Miraculously, the plans came together. It was certainly far from the start of high school I had hoped for her, but it would work.

When we realized Blaine would not be able to come home for the next few months, we decided Kaci and Kamryn should fly down to see him, and my final goal during this trip home was to get that booked. We knew Blaine's white count would only be high enough to be around extra people during week three of his chemo cycle. Between his restrictions and the girls' schedules, and the fact there were only limited flights on the affordable airline out of Springfield, finding a time that worked was no easy task! We did finally settle on an acceptable date, and I bought their tickets. Blaine was going to be so excited to see them! We tried to fly Kaia down also, but between her classes and practice schedule, she just could not get away.

I had barely started to adjust to being home when it was time to return to Texas. I hugged the girls one last time, and my friend, Carolyn, drove me to the airport. The last time I had made this trip, I was sure Blaine and I would both be home in two weeks. This time I had absolutely no idea when we would be back. I was slowly adjusting to the realization I had no actual control over anything, but I still wanted to at least have a plan. Now I had neither. I had said goodbye to the girls and chatted with Carolyn as we drove as if everything were fine, but inside I was struggling with the sensation I was drowning. Dark waves of fear were constantly threatening to close over me, and I was using every ounce of strength I had to keep them down.

Because my mother was very sick while I was growing up, my childhood had always been unpredictable, and adult responsibilities were mine much earlier than they should have been. My most important priority had always been to build a close family with children who felt secure and knew their parents were there for them. Now, we had left Kamryn to basically raise herself and Kaci with the stress of maintaining our home and ensuring her little sister had what she needed. I loved them so much, and I desperately did not want this to be their story. My sister pointed out to me that we hadn't abandoned them and that I was still very much a part of their lives emotionally. I talked with them every day and did my very best to be involved, but it wasn't the same as being there, and we both knew it. Deep down, I knew God was in control and He would use this to shape them to become the people He wanted them to be, but I really wished this didn't have to be their story.

Chapter 22

As much as I missed the girls, it felt right to be back with Blaine. He had been feeling pretty good when I left, but now he seemed almost normal again. We were watching a movie the night I got back, and I kept noticing an odd smell. I just couldn't quite identify it. "I keep thinking I'm smelling something, but I can't quite figure it out. It smells like brownies."

"It's cougar poop," Blaine replied. I laughed out loud. He said the weirdest things sometimes! "No. I'm serious. Mike put cougar poop in the attic to get the racoons to leave."

Cougar poop! Things were escalating here quickly! I already suspected this whole experience would change my life. Now I was sure of it. I would certainly never feel the same about brownies again.

The next day was a busy one. Blaine had lab work, a chest X-ray, and the first MRI of his arm since he started the chemo. He had an advantage over most cancer patients in the fact that we could see part of Lumpy, and we could already tell it was shrinking. Almost every day it seemed to be a little bit smaller, and it had turned from a bright pink/purple color to solid black. I couldn't wait to get the MRI results. I just knew they would show it was dead, and I assumed that meant he could be done with the chemo.

We didn't have to wait long. One of the amazing things about MD Anderson is how quickly the doctors have access to the test results. Blaine had an appointment with Dr. Baldyga that afternoon. She walked in absolutely beaming. "Mr. and Mrs. Parker! We have such good news for you!" She pulled up the images on her computer from his last MRI right before he started the chemo next to his images from that day. We could very clearly see that the tumor was *significantly* smaller than it had been. Maybe even more important than its size, the report said the "internal enhancement has dramatically diminished," meaning the cancer cells were dying.

This is what we had been praying for! I was so excited. "That means we can stop the chemo then, right?"

"Oh, of course not! It's clearly working. Why would we stop?" She went on to explain to me, again, that the purpose of the chemo was not even necessarily to treat the tumor on Blaine's arm. She was trying to kill any random cells that may be making their way to his lungs. The fact that the chemo was so effective in killing Lumpy meant it was likely also very effective in killing the more worrisome cells, if there were any. That made sense to me, but I was so disappointed. I wanted so badly for him to be done. Regardless, those images on the computer screen were remarkable, and it was such a good feeling to know the awful chemo was actually accomplishing something.

We talked about plans for the next round of chemo, which would start in the morning. She prescribed baclofen, which would hopefully eliminate the hiccups, and put in orders for a few days of IV fluids to go through his pump after the chemo was finished in an effort to prevent the dehydration. Blaine wasn't thrilled with having to carry the pump around longer than necessary but agreed it would be better than having to go back to the ER. As worried as I was about him starting another cycle, I left Dr. Baldyga's office feeling like we had a good plan in place and optimistic that this cycle would be easier for him.

The next few days went by pretty uneventfully. By now, we knew what to expect, and the whole process was much less terrifying. He actually felt pretty good through the days he received the chemo. The hiccups even stayed away until the third day. Unfortunately, at that point, they were so violent he shook the whole car! They didn't last long, though, and we were making our way through the week surprisingly easily. On his second to last day of the infusions, he was scheduled to be in a different building. They did this every now and then, and we never knew why, but we appreciated the change of scenery.

Blaine fell asleep while the chemo was running, so I decided to take a walk. Although we weren't in that building often, I felt comfortable there and had a good understanding of the general layout. I didn't like walking past patients receiving their treatment. Most kept their doors closed, but some didn't, and it always made me feel awkward, so I headed for the first exit door I saw. Looking back on this now, I vaguely remember there being a sign on the door I probably should have paid attention to, but I just walked on through. The door shut, and locked, and I found myself in some sort of a storage area. No problem. I knew the general direction to the elevators, so I started walking. Weirdly, there were no elevators where I was expecting them to be, but there were stairs. I would just walk down a flight and come out on the next floor and find the elevator.

I opened the door to the stairwell, jogged down the stairs and reached to open the door. It was locked! What in the world? I jogged down the next flight. Surely that one would be open. Nope. Locked. There was no choice but to keep going. I had started on the eighth floor. I checked the door on each level, fully expecting it to open. Each door was locked. When I finally reached the bottom floor and realized that one was locked also, I knew I had a problem. I had gotten myself locked in! The air in the stairwell became thinner as I realized I was trapped.

Thankfully, there was a sign on the door with the number to call hospital security if you had a problem, leading me to believe I was not the only caregiver dumb enough to get locked in. Knowing I wasn't the only one didn't help. I took a big gulp of air as I dialed the number. "Hello, MD Anderson security. Do you have an emergency?"

I felt like an idiot. "No. I am just locked in a stairwell."

"Are you a patient?"

"No, my husband is." He asked what building I was in and instructed me to look through the window and describe what I saw so they could find me. The lights were all off in the room on the other side, and it seemed to be some sort of art museum. Where on earth had I gone? The security guard told me someone would be there soon to let me out and I should call back if I needed anything before he got there.

Thankfully, he got there soon because I just knew the walls were closing in. I remembered the raccoons being trapped in our attic. Fortunately, I kept my cool enough not to run around destroying things. When the guard let me out, I thanked him and pointed out having all those doors locked was really a safety issue. Surely I wouldn't be the only person who might walk through the wrong door. He then pointed out I could have simply gone through the door that led to the outside. After he said that, I remembered there being another door. I had sped right past it. Oh, brother! I really was losing it.

The guard led me back to the main elevators. I decided I had had enough exercise—and humiliation—for the day and just went back to Blaine's room. He had woken up and was glad to see me. "Where have you been?"

"You are not going to believe this." I told him the story and he thought it was hilarious. He was the one who was supposed to have chemo brain!

Chapter 23

Other than my stairwell incident, the infusion part of cycle three went very well, and just like that, we were halfway through the planned six cycles! When the chemo infusions were completed, they sent Blaine home with three liters of fluid to run through his CVC line every night. He hated lugging it around when it was full, but he felt better through this cycle than any of the others. I was sure we had turned a corner, that we had found the perfect combination of treatments, and the rest of the cycles would go easily.

Throughout all this time, Mike continued to try to solve the raccoon problem. Nothing worked. They were quite happy in their home, and there was no way we were going to convince them to leave. Finally, he decided he just needed to trap them. He brought a big cage and carried it through the door in our bedroom, along with a bag of marshmallows he was positive would entice them into the cage. He set the marshmallows down and turned for a second to get the cage set. I saw a flash of black as a baby raccoon scampered away with the entire bag of marshmallows! Mike groaned and came back down to get another bag while I stood at the bottom of the ladder trying to stifle my giggles. He finally got everything set in the attic and told us he would return in the morning to relocate the raccoons he had caught.

Sometime in the middle of the night, we heard the cage door slam shut. His plan had worked! We braced ourselves for the angry raccoon noises we were sure would come, but instead, we heard them peacefully walking all around the attic. We learned the next morning one of them had been able to get the marshmallows without getting caught in the trap. Those raccoons were smart! Lydia apologized over and over to us, but truthfully, we didn't mind at all. What would entertain us if they ever actually did get rid of them?

Blaine had made it through the first eight days of the chemo cycle without any trouble. We had been warned days four through seven are typically the worst, but he had sailed right through those without any problems. The extra fluid had really done the trick! On day number nine, though, he got up and just seemed . . . off. He slept a little more than he had been, and when he was awake, he was strangely quiet. When he did talk, he was . . . mean. Every word out of his mouth was hateful. I didn't quite know what to make of it, but honestly, if anyone had a right to be in a bad mood, it was him. He couldn't get comfortable in any of the chairs, and I was thankful when he finally just went back to bed, hopeful he would wake up in a better mood tomorrow.

He didn't. I completely understood why he would feel depressed and crabby, but the change had been so sudden. He went to bed one night and was a totally different person when he woke up. We went in that morning for labs and then came back to the Cottage. Blaine alternated between trying to work and trying to nap. He barely spoke all day, which I preferred because when he did talk, it was only to complain.

A few hours later, Dr. Baldyga's nurse called to go over his labs with me. They only called if they were concerned about something, and as expected, his numbers weren't good. His kidney function was much better, thanks to the extra fluid, but his white count, hemoglobin, and platelets were all very low. All of that was bad, but most concerning was his neutrophil Abs. This was the number that indicated how susceptible he would be to an infection. His value was 0.09. I knew absolutely nothing about a neutrophil Abs reading, but I knew anything that started with 0.0 could not be good. She asked me how he was feeling.

I didn't really know how to answer her. Blaine was asleep in the other room, so I tried to explain his change in mood. "He doesn't seem to feel awful physically, but he's become so . . . crabby." I knew that sounded stupid. Of course the man was crabby! Who wouldn't be crabby in his situation? "He's just not normally crabby. It's strange because he's just acting so differently. Of course, I guess that's to be expected, right?" I was floundering. I didn't know how to explain it.

"Please keep a close eye on him and call us if there are any changes." She paused and then went on. "Christi, I know you understand he absolutely cannot be exposed to any germs, but with his platelet count being so low, you also have to make sure he does not get any cuts or have any falls. Even just bumping into something could be very dangerous because his blood will not be able to clot."

I sighed. Something new to worry about. I thanked her for calling, promised to keep her updated, and went back to my day.

While Blaine and I were dealing with all of this, back home in our real world, Kamryn was starting school. Every other year of our daughters' lives, we had made a big deal of the first day of school. Tears stung my eyes when Kaci sent me her little sister's first day of school picture. I had left Kamryn with clear directions, and she and I Face-Timed for the classes for which she needed teacher involvement. It wasn't seamless, but it worked, and although I was sad not to be there with her, overall, I think we were both satisfied with the first day.

Blaine continued trying to work while I was helping Kamryn, but he was having more and more trouble finding a comfortable way to sit. We didn't think much about it, but it certainly wasn't helping his mood. A little while later, he came out of the bathroom and looked even more pale than his new usual. "Are you okay?" I asked.

"Yes. It just really hurt when I went to the bathroom. Stop asking me about everything. I'm sure it's nothing."

A couple hours later, he came out of the bathroom again, but now all of the color had drained from his face, and he was shaking.

"Are you sure you're okay?"

"I'm fine. I went to the bathroom, and it was the worst pain I've ever had in my life, but I'm fine."

At that point, he gave up the idea of trying to work and just went to bed. I had never seen him look like that. He insisted he was fine, but I knew something wasn't right. I had promised to keep the nurse updated, so I sent her a message via his online portal.

My phone rang ten minutes later. She wanted to know all about his pain. I felt so awkward talking to her about it, and I knew Blaine was listening from the bedroom. We often have different opinions about what is concerning and what isn't, and he frequently thinks I make a bigger deal out of medical issues than necessary, so I was working very hard not to do that. Honestly, I played things down a bit to keep him happy and because I felt almost like I was betraying him to talk about something so personal.

"Is there any chance his pain is actually like a mouth sore?" I asked.

"Yes. I'm sure that's what it is. Patients receiving chemotherapy can get mouth sores anywhere along their digestive tract." She paused. "You need to bring him into the emergency room." That is exactly the opposite of what I was hoping to hear. I knew he was going to be mad.

"Do you think that's absolutely necessary? He doesn't have a fever, and he's really not going to want to go."

"I think he needs to, but Dr. Baldyga is already gone for the day. I will contact the on-call physician and see what he thinks, but my advice to you is that you just go ahead and take him."

I hung up the phone and walked into the bedroom. Sure enough, Blaine had heard the whole conversation. He was perched on the edge of the bed, his hands balled into tight fists. "Why did you lie to her? You just want drama. I'm fine. You exaggerate everything!"

I took a deep, steadying breath as he continued to spew accusations. He went on and on while I just stood and took it. His words should have crushed me, but instead they seemed to bounce right off. Somehow God had given me an extra layer of protection, allowing me to see his reaction for what it was and not take it personally.

He finally ran out of complaints. "I'm not going to the ER."

"Okay, but it is time to get the pump taken off." His last bag of fluid was almost finished, and it was time to leave for his appointment to have it unhooked.

The drive to the hospital was a quiet one. He was steaming. I was scared. Just as we were about to turn into the parking garage, Dr. Simmons, the on-call sarcoma oncologist, called. He was encouraging me to take Blaine to the ER immediately instead of just going to get his pump unhooked.

"I'm not really sure he needs to go to the ER. He says he doesn't feel that bad, and he really does not want to go."

"The rectal pain he is having could be a medical emergency."

"But he's not even running a fever."

He was quiet for a moment and then said, "Christi, his white count is so low that his body most likely does not even have the resources to raise his temperature. He needs to go to the ER now."

His words settled over me. I knew that was really bad. I was terrified Blaine would still insist he was not going, but when I told him what the doctor had said, the fight went out of him, and he agreed. I made a sharp turn away from the parking garage and toward the ER and dropped Blaine off at the door. I couldn't believe we were back here again!

Chapter 24

I suspect Dr. Simmons had called the ER to let them know we were coming, even though I hadn't agreed, because in the few minutes it took me to park the car and walk back inside, they had already gotten Blaine into a room and were swooping in like a pit crew at a racetrack. There were at least six staff in his room, and each of them was rushing to complete their specific task. It was really impressive! It was also really scary. They certainly hadn't acted like that during his previous visits. A dull throbbing began in the back of my head. Before I knew it, they had started two different kinds of IV antibiotics and were rushing him out for an MRI.

A few minutes later, the doctor came back in to talk to me. "We suspect your husband has a rectal abscess. If the MRI confirms our suspicions, he will need emergency surgery, and with his current white count and platelet count, this will be very dangerous. We will let you know as soon as we know for sure."

She hurried out to take care of her other patients. I began praying like crazy and texting those closest to Blaine with the new update. All day long I had been haunted by the significance of the day. Exactly twenty-four years earlier, Blaine's mother had passed away following a very short fight with cancer after she had been misdiagnosed, exactly like Blaine had been. I couldn't believe that on the anniversary of the end of her life, Blaine was fighting for his. To make matters even worse, she was only fifty years old when she died, and Blaine had just turned fifty. I hadn't breathed a word of this to anyone, but I finally broke down and told his friend Chris. He took a long time to reply. Finally, my phone chimed. "He is not going to die tonight. He is not." That's all it said, and although I knew he had no way of knowing for sure, somehow it made me feel better.

Before long, they brought Blaine back to the room, and soon after that, the doctor came to tell us the MRI had actually not shown an abscess! He did not need surgery, but he was still very sick. His white count was now down to 0.2, and his hemoglobin was dangerously low. Even though blood was in very short supply at the hospital, they were going to give Blaine two units and then admit him to the hospital for continued IV antibiotics and monitoring.

Everyone who was admitted to the hospital had to have a COVID test first. This time, Blaine didn't laugh! The tech who came in to do the test was not taking any chances on not getting an accurate sample and jammed the stick way up his nose. It really hurt him, but I was the one who had to blink back tears. I knew he felt awful. Adding a painful COVID test to his trouble felt like more than either of us could handle.

It took a long time for the blood to be delivered to his room, but eventually it arrived, and the nurse hooked it to his CVC line. "You are more than welcome to stay while he receives his transfusion, but once we take him upstairs, you will have to leave."

I just stared at her, blinking slowly as my mind tried to process what she had said. "Why can't I stay with him?"

"It is against the rules now because of COVID. Only patients who do not speak English, are completely mentally incapacitated, or are very near death are allowed to have a caregiver stay with them. The nurses will do their best to keep you updated on his condition and will let you know when you can come take him home."

The throbbing in my head grew stronger. I was thrilled to hear Blaine didn't meet those qualifications, but I couldn't leave him. Fortunately, by the time they were ready to move him upstairs, he had a different nurse. I decided to take a chance. "Can I go with him?"

She gave me a sympathetic smile. "Sure." She glanced around and then lowered her voice. "It's a little touchy. The rules are changing every day. No one ever knows what's going on, so just act like you're supposed to be there, and chances are no one will question you. If you leave his room, however, someone will probably notice and not let you back in, so I suggest you just stay there." I grinned my thanks and fought the urge to hug her. I could do that! I could do whatever I needed to do. I just didn't want to have to leave him there alone.

It was sometime in the early morning hours when they finally moved him to an actual hospital room. I was surprised, and thankful, to see there was a small couch. His new nurse even gave me a little blanket and a pillow, and I lay down to try to get some sleep. It was not easy. My mind was still racing from all that had happened that day, and while I was thankful for the blanket, it did little to combat the freezing temperature in the hospital. My exhaustion was stronger than the circumstances, though, and I soon began to doze off.

Beep! My eyes flew open. *Beep, beep, beep, beep!* Something was wrong with the IV. So much for my idea of sleeping. Thankfully, the nurse happened to be walking by his door and came in to check it.

She pushed a few buttons and the beeping stopped. "No problem! Your vancomycin is finished. Go back to sleep."

I lay back down and closed my eyes for what seemed like a second. *Beep! Beep, beep, beep, beep!*

I sat back up. It was going to be a long night. *Beep, beep, beep, beep!* Blaine and I stared at each other. The beeping continued, but no one came to fix it. Finally, I pushed the call button.

"Can I help you?" came a mysterious voice.

"My husband's IV is beeping again."

"Okay. Just a moment."

A few minutes later a different nurse came in and pushed a few buttons. "No problem! Just an air bubble."

This scenario repeated itself over and over and over. In addition to regular fluid, Blaine was receiving multiple other intravenous medications. Whenever one of them finished or got an air bubble, it would beep. Sometimes more than one line would have an issue at the same time, and they would each beep at a different time and a different pitch. *Beep, beep . . . beep . . . beep-beep!* Sometimes, the nurses would catch it fairly quickly, but usually no one would hear it. Blaine didn't like to bother them, and somehow he barely noticed the beeping, but it drove me completely batty.

I finally gave up trying to sleep when the sun came up a couple hours later. I hadn't eaten since lunch the previous day and was completely starving, but I knew I couldn't leave the room. Thankfully, MD Anderson has an excellent food service, and I was able to call and order breakfast for both of us. I placed the order and then sat next to Blaine on the bed. When I got up a few minutes later, lights flashed and an automated voice commanded "Don't get up! Don't get up!" Soon the nurse came rushing into the room.

"Mr. Parker, do you need something? You are not allowed to get out of bed by yourself!" We quickly explained it was just me. She laughed and turned off the alarm. Blaine, however, was pretty indignant that he wasn't allowed to get out of bed without notifying them. The nurse explained that the bed alarm is normal protocol for any patient who has had a blood transfusion because they might be unsteady on their feet, but in Blaine's case in particular they were worried that if he fell, he would be in real danger because his platelets were so low. He didn't care. He can be quite persuasive when he wants to be, and he somehow convinced her to disengage the system.

The rest of the day went by pretty uneventfully. Thankfully, I had thought to throw the phone charger into my bag before I left the Cottage.

I really wished I had thought to put on more comfortable clothes and pack a toothbrush, but I survived.

Blaine slept most of the day while I scrolled aimlessly through Facebook and daydreamed about the girls' upcoming visit. Kaci and Kamryn were supposed to be flying down in three days. I couldn't wait to see them, but slowly the realization that Blaine was likely to still be pretty sick set in. Tears slid down my face as I imagined how they would feel seeing their dad like this, and I knew I couldn't put them through that. I called the airline and rescheduled the tickets for later in the week. It broke my heart, but there was no choice. I could wait a few more days.

I made it through the whole day, but that evening someone in charge finally discovered I was there. I had to go. Blaine did seem a little stronger to me by then, but it was still so hard to leave him! Begrudgingly, I grabbed my bag and glanced out the window as I went to kiss him goodbye. I sucked in my breath as I took in the unexpected view. The sky was brilliant shades of orange, and the monstrous buildings glowed as the light reflected off their metal sides. When I think of sunsets, nature images come to mind—the sun setting behind mountains, trees, or open fields—but now I was watching it set behind a sea of hospitals, and I was completely amazed to discover it was still beautiful. It was a lovely reminder that God was there, and He hadn't changed. Our life was completely different, but the sunset Creator was the same.

I walked into the Cottage and headed straight for bed. My entire body ached. I listened to the raccoons walking around above me and couldn't quite decide if the sound was comforting or scary. They definitely seemed bigger now that I was alone. They must have sounded comforting because I fell asleep almost instantly and slept straight through the night. The restful night was such a gift because I rarely slept well, and that night I had so much on my mind. Once again, life or death decisions needed to be made, and I needed to be well-rested so I could think clearly.

Chapter 25

I called to check on Blaine first thing the next morning. He said he hadn't gotten much sleep but felt okay. He almost always said he felt okay, so this meant nothing to me. They had already drawn labs, but the results weren't posted yet, and he hadn't seen Dr. Baldyga. It was so frustrating not to be there to talk to her. In my mind, the chemo needed to stop. We had physical evidence that it was working very effectively against the cancer cells that had formed Lumpy. Surely, if there were any random cells floating around inside his body, they would have been completely obliterated. It just didn't make sense to me to keep subjecting his body to this poison if the cancer was already dead.

On the other hand, I was very aware of how much I didn't know. MD Anderson has the highest success rate of curing sarcoma of anywhere in the whole world. I really had no choice but to trust what they said, but trusting does not come easily for me. I knew there was a specific protocol they followed. If a patient had a sarcoma, they gave six cycles of chemo. Research had proven that was the most effective treatment, but did that mean it was the most effective treatment specifically for Blaine? I, of course, had no way of knowing. I was terrified we would stop the chemo prematurely and the sarcoma cells would form in his lungs, but I was also terrified he would take more chemo and somehow that would kill him. There was simply no option but to pray hard and trust the doctors.

A few hours later, Blaine called to let me know he was being released from the hospital. I wasn't sure they didn't just need his bed, but I was glad he would be back home. I quickly drove to the hospital to get him. The nurses had told me to come to the room so I could help him get to the car, but somehow they failed to notify the COVID guards at the door. Breaking into that hospital without having an actual patient with you was no easy task! Those people took their jobs very seriously.

After multiple calls to the floor, they finally let me past them, and I went up to help Blaine carry the truckload of things they were sending home with him. I signed a form promising I would be driving, and then we just walked out. I was totally surprised by this, and frankly, a little annoyed. He was really sick, and it was a long walk from his room to the car. I had expected a nurse to wheel him out like every other hospital dismissal I had ever been a part of, but that's not how it worked. The nurses here were so busy. They really needed to be able to focus all their attention on their patients who were too sick to go home.

The elevator opened, and we stepped in with a few other people. As we were descending, suddenly panic swept over Blaine's face. I took one look at him and somehow knew what had happened. He had lost control of his bowels right there in the elevator. Fortunately, there were no outward indications and no one else could tell, but I knew Blaine was completely mortified anyway. We finally got to the ground floor and headed straight for the restroom so he could clean up. In every stall in every restroom at MD Anderson, there is a sign with a number to call if you have soiled yourself and need a change of clothes, so this must be a pretty common issue, but somehow I was still totally unprepared for this. I knew Blaine was horrified, and I felt so bad for him. As we had done over and over again, we just kept going. He cleaned himself up as best he could, and I went to get the car. Surely this would be a one-time issue.

It wasn't. The issue continued. It actually got worse. Twice that night, he got up thinking he just needed to urinate, but as soon as he stood up … I'll spare you the details, but let's just say, it was a rough night. It got so bad that he never knew what would happen when he moved. Of course, he still had the rectal sores, so on top of its being embarrassing for him, it was also horribly painful physically. This obviously was a problem even if we were alone at the Cottage, but he needed to go in to have labs done that morning. How on earth was he supposed to go out in public?

I was sitting at my computer trying to finish a little work when he shuffled in. "Christi, I think I need you to get me some adult diapers."

"Okay." I wanted to cry but held it together. He looked so miserable, it made my heart physically ache. He went back to bed, and I messaged Dr. Baldyga's office asking for help. He couldn't live like this. They had to do something to fix it. This is an actual line from that message: "I am on my way to the store to buy my big, strong, fiercely independent husband adult diapers so he can go get labs to see if he has any white count left in the middle of a pandemic." I re-read the message before I hit send and shook my head. I just couldn't believe this was our life!

The nurse didn't have much of a response to my pathetic message but advised me to increase the Imodium he was already taking for diarrhea. I was expecting something fancier and felt a little dumb for not thinking of that myself. I headed to the store to stock up on Imodium and to make my first ever purchase of adult diapers. My hands trembled slightly as I pulled the box off the shelf, and I fought the desire to look around to see if anyone was watching me. When I forced myself to really examine the box, relief washed over me. They didn't look like diapers at all. They almost looked like regular underwear! Blaine was even happy with them. It certainly wasn't cool to be wearing disposable underwear, but it wasn't as bad as he had been expecting, and they certainly made things less stressful.

As if our lives weren't dramatic enough, the next morning I woke up to a post on Blaine's Facebook group from a friend who follows the weather very closely. There was a hurricane headed for Houston! I had to read the post twice to make sure I was understanding it correctly. I was. There was a hurricane coming. Lydia had told us stories about living through Hurricane Harvey a few years earlier, about how the Cottage had flooded badly.

In the back of my mind, I knew we were heading into hurricane season, but I assumed we wouldn't have any issues. I had always been taught God doesn't give you more than you can handle. I was pretty confident I could not handle a hurricane. I had felt for months that my life had been hit by a hurricane, and now there was a literal one headed straight for me! We were about forty minutes from the coast, but the report was predicting widespread wind damage well inland. It wasn't expected to make landfall for a few days, but soon all of the news reports were advising people to prepare. Lydia brought us flashlights and batteries and cases of water and advised us to pay close attention to the weather.

This is the point when I started to worry I might lose it. I wasn't actually afraid of the hurricane; I had been through a hurricane before. It was that there was now *one more thing* I had to pay close attention to. I had to pay attention to all of Blaine's random symptoms, all of his medications, his temperature, his bowel movements, Kamryn's school and general life, Kaci's life, Kaia's life, my work, the bills; the list went on and on and on, and now I had to add a hurricane to it? What happened to the idea that God wouldn't give me more than I could handle?

To make matters even worse, I realized the girls should not be here. Blaine was actually sicker now than he was when I took him to the hospital. I absolutely did not want them to have to carry the image of him like this in their minds for the rest of their lives. His white count was also not rebounding the way Dr. Baldyga had anticipated, so he would still not be able to fight any random germs they might bring with them. We just couldn't risk his being exposed to anyone new. And, of course, there was a hurricane coming. Who knew what that would do to the flight schedules? I did not want them trapped at an airport somewhere. This, really, I think is what I was afraid would break me. I had the strength to keep moving through this awful experience because I knew Kaci and Kamryn would be with us soon. Now they wouldn't, and I would have to continue on my own. My heart was breaking, but there was no choice. I canceled their flight.

Chapter 26

Thankfully, for us anyway, the hurricane changed direction and didn't affect Houston at all, and as the doctors had predicted, Blaine did eventually start to feel better. Both situations I had been so worried about had either not been an issue after all or had been temporary and survivable. I know the vast majority of things I stress about end up falling into one of these two categories. If I could just learn not to be stressed about them in the first place, my life would be a lot easier.

Blaine continued to need his labs checked every day because his counts stayed so low, but soon he seemed strong enough that I was reasonably comfortable dropping him off. I went to my McDonald's to wait for his text telling me he was finished. Instead, his text said, "My nose is bleeding." I sucked in my breath as my heart pounded. Two months ago a message like that wouldn't have meant anything serious, but now it was a potential emergency. I knew I wouldn't be allowed into the hospital without him so there was nothing to do but sit and wait. Thankfully, the bleeding stopped, and he was able to go back to the Cottage with me.

He actually felt pretty decent and was up working, so we were shocked when Dr. Baldyga's nurse called an hour later. "Hi, Veronica!" I kept my voice happy and light, hoping to magically influence any bad news she might have for me.

"Hi, Christi. I'm afraid I have some bad news about Blaine's labs." So much for my happy-voice effort. "His platelets are down to 9." I swallowed hard. I knew a normal platelet count was between 140 and 440. Having a count of 9 was just inconceivable to me. "He needs a transfusion imme-diately. They're expecting him in the ATC." She paused before going on. "And Christi, don't let him bump into anything."

I thanked her and assured her we were heading that way. Blaine had been watching me while I talked. He let out a huge sigh and got up to put his shoes on without even knowing what he needed. Thankfully, the ATC was able to get him in quickly, and the entire ordeal only took about an hour. Blaine really was feeling shockingly good for someone walking around with almost no platelets, but hopefully the transfusion would help him feel even better.[9]

I was working later that afternoon when Kamryn called. "Mom! Zach just invited me to his homecoming dance!"

My heart flip-flopped. "That's wonderful, Kam!" Part of me was so happy. Part of me was so unhappy.

She went on to tell me all about their plans and how she and Kaci were going to go shopping that weekend for a dress. I was so excited for her, but I couldn't believe I was missing our last daughter's first dance! I would miss all of it—the shopping, the planning, the getting ready, the waiting up to hear the report when she got home. It was so unfair! I fought hard to keep my voice from cracking so Kamryn wouldn't realize I was anything but thrilled, and I focused on soaking in all of her joy. When the conversation was over though, I walked outside so Blaine wouldn't see. And then I cried.

The next morning, Blaine and I headed back to the hospital for his daily lab check. For those patients unlucky enough to need labs drawn on the weekends, the hospital handles things differently. Instead of sending patients home while a nurse looks over the results, they are required to stay and have the results reviewed in person. We knew this might involve a significant wait, so I stayed to keep him company.

By this point, Blaine was on a first-name basis with all of the nurses who drew his blood. (Because he had the CVC line, it had to be drawn by a nurse instead of a phlebotomist). There are always significantly fewer patients waiting for labs on the weekends than Monday through Friday, so we didn't have to wait long, and he actually got in with his favorite nurse, Mara.

"Good morning, Mr. and Mrs. Parker! How are you today?" We both loved Mara. She was surrounded every single day by unhappy, sometimes dying, people, but joy seemed to ooze out of her. We always left the lab feeling a little lighter on the days she was Blaine's nurse. Every time we saw her, she literally giggled at some point during our interaction. Today, she didn't giggle. No matter what she did, his blood would not come out. "Your line is clogged. Have you gotten a platelet transfusion lately?"

"Yes, I had one yesterday."

"Ohhhhhh . . . that makes sense then. Platelets are very, very sticky. Every time you get one, you need to ask your nurse to flush the line at least twice. That will help it not to get clogged. Unfortunately, this one is completely blocked. You're going to have to go to the vascular department and see if they can fix it." Thankfully, she was able to draw his blood through the other line, but we still needed to go to our most hated place in the hospital, where we knew we might be waiting for hours.

It did take a while for Blaine to be called back to a room, but it wasn't as bad as we were fearing. The nurse confirmed the line was clogged completely but thought it would be easily fixed. He reiterated to us that if Blaine were to ever receive a platelet transfusion again, we must ask them to flush it a few extra times. He injected medicine into the line and told us to come back in an hour to see if it had dissolved the clog. We went down to the cafeteria to grab some lunch while we waited.

Thankfully, after an hour, the line was cleared. When the nurse went to flush the other line, however, he discovered it was now clogged! We were pretty concerned by this, but he assured us it's not uncommon. He injected the medicine into the second line, and we went to sit in the waiting room. The nurse called us back an hour later and confirmed the second line was now clear.

We were finally free to go wait for the nurse to review Blaine's lab results with us. We knew that could take a long time too. This is certainly not how we had hoped to spend our Saturday. Oddly though, neither of us really cared that much. In our normal life, having our day so totally interrupted and waiting for hours and hours would have been infuriating. Now, somehow, it was just life. We were learning to roll with whatever happened. We were together. Blaine didn't feel awful. Little irritations didn't matter as much as they did before.

Eventually, Blaine's name was called, and we went back to meet with the nurse. "Good news! Your blood counts are all better than yesterday!"

"Great! Does that mean we don't need to come in tomorrow?"

"Oh no. They're still very low. We definitely need to check them again."

We thanked her and grabbed our things. We didn't get the results we were hoping for, but better was better, and we chose to focus on the win.

Chapter 27

The next few days crept by without much excitement. I loved those kinds of days! Although Blaine's platelets rebounded very slowly, they finally reached the level where he could return to his twice-a-week lab schedule. He didn't have much energy, but all things considered, he didn't seem to feel nearly as bad as you would expect with those numbers. He was able to work most days as long as he could take a nap or two throughout the day. Thankfully, his office was now about six feet from our bedroom, so that was easy. He lay down to take a nap one day, and I made a quick run to pick up some groceries.

I was surprised to see he was already up again when I returned. "How was your nap?"

He laughed. "Not great. It was really hot in our room. I noticed the vent was closed so I got up to open it and then lay back down. I was just about to close my eyes when I saw a little raccoon hand reach down and close the vent again!"

"I can't believe I missed that. They're so adorable!"

He gave me a look. "Not adorable. I got up and opened it, but as soon as I climbed back in bed, the little bugger did it again!"

"Oh." I still thought they were adorable but knew Blaine wouldn't appreciate my opinion.

"This time I got up and opened it again and then just stood off to the side. When he stuck his hand through, I touched him gently with a water bottle and yelled at him."

This time I gave him a look.

"I did feel bad, but they've got to leave the vents alone!"

He was right, of course, but I was still sad I had missed it. Those guys really were the best entertainment!

Not so entertaining was the fact that pieces of insulation kept appearing all over the kitchen bar and in other random places through the Cottage. It didn't take long to realize what was happening. The racoons were throwing it down through the vents. I had kept the Facebook group updated on the racoon shenanigans, and someone suggested they were probably telling stories about the humans who wouldn't leave. We decided she was probably right, but we were determined to stay. We made a point not to leave any food on the bar, swept up the insulation every morning, and just went on our merry way. We were determined to win this turf war.

The insulation issue was irritating, but somehow having a conflict like that was kind of . . . nice. It felt good to solve a problem just by moving our food or doing a little sweeping. Unfortunately, the time for our next real battle, the fourth chemotherapy infusion cycle, was about to begin. I so desperately wanted time to speed up so we could go home to our girls and our real life, but I was terrified for Blaine to go through it again, and I wanted time to slow down so he didn't have to do it. This feeling of wanting two polar opposite situations simultaneously was something I was learning to live with, but it constantly made me feel a little crazy. At this point though, the terror of putting him through the chemo again was winning, and in my desire to slow time down, I did what any logical person would do: I stayed up super late. If I didn't go to bed, the morning wouldn't come, right?

Wrong. Of course, it came anyway. Blaine was scheduled for labs, a chest X-ray to make sure his CVC lines were still in place, and an appointment to meet with the oncologist to go over the plan for this cycle. Two days earlier, his platelets had only been at 44. They must be at least 100, or they would have to delay the treatment. A delay meant we would have to stay in Houston longer, but his safety was clearly the priority. He had his labs drawn and the chest X-ray, and we went to wait for Dr. Baldyga to give us the results.

She walked in smiling. "Mr. Parker, your platelets are up to 102!" He was always such an overachiever! We talked about how the last cycle had gone, and she asked if we had any questions.

"Actually, I do have a question. This spot has come up on my shoulder. Do you think it's anything to be concerned about?"

"I'm also a little worried about that spot on his face," I added. Now that all of his facial hair was gone, there was an oddly shaped, brown freckle on his jawline that I had never seen before.

Dr. Baldyga looked at both spots. "Yes, we probably need to have those checked out." She asked Veronica to make Blaine an appointment with a dermatologist at the hospital. I had been expecting her to tell us they were nothing and then I would feel silly for worrying. Now I had a brand-new problem to obsess about.

Interestingly though, I didn't. I wish I could say I just trusted God, but that wasn't really true. I think I was just learning to compartmentalize different areas of concern. It was like I wrapped them in a box and put them in a different part of my mind until they had to be dealt with. Every now and then some worry would start to leak out of its container, but I would stuff it back in so I could deal with the biggest issue in front of me. I'm not positive a psychologist would say this was particularly healthy, but it did help me get through this crazy time.

Even with the new skin cancer concern, when we left her office, I felt much braver. For the fourth round of chemo, they would keep the treatments we knew worked, the baclofen to help with the hiccups and the extra fluid to keep him hydrated. In addition, this time they were going to start him on antibiotics as soon as the chemo infusions were completed to give him some extra protection when his white count tanked. I knew we had a big God and He had given us good medicine and smart doctors. Plus, Blaine was now on the downhill side of this. We were going to be okay.

The next four days of chemo infusions went by easily. He had one four-hour stretch of horrendous hiccups, but those were the worst of his symptoms. He felt pretty good overall, and we were so much more comfortable now with the whole process. Somehow during this week, Labor Day came and went. I couldn't believe we had missed the entire summer! For Blaine and me, time had stopped, but somehow for the rest of the world it just kept marching on. At home, people were going on with their lives. Our friends had gone on vacations, spent days at the pool, and had months of relaxed family time. None of that seemed real. I felt like I was dreaming those things had happened, or maybe I was dreaming our life in Houston was happening. I felt dizzy when I allowed myself to think about it, like I was standing on the edge of some sort of portal, one foot on either side, in two different worlds.

Day five arrived, the last day of the infusion. The only thing left to do was go back to the ATC that evening to have the red devil bag taken off, and then they would start him on the fluid. I was relieved the fluid was coming because Blaine slept *all* day. It was good he was getting rest, but his not waking up made me nervous. I had learned from earlier cycles this probably meant he was dehydrated. Sure enough, when I finally woke him up and we went in to have the pump changed, they discovered his heart rate was very elevated—another sign of dehydration. No one worried about this too much as they were hooking him up to a three-liter bag of fluid, but he continued to sleep for the next three days. I woke him up to take his medicine and when it was time to get his bag replenished, but other than that, he pretty much just stayed asleep. Dr. Baldyga's staff confirmed it was normal to be exhausted by this point in the treatment, and they were happy he was able to rest as well as he was. He had also started talking less and less when he was awake. He would answer questions, but that was all. It was extra lonely for me, but I worked a lot and watched some TV. In my normal life, I hardly ever had time to sit and just watch TV. Now, I suddenly had too much time.

I had kept up pretty well with Elesha, the woman who stayed with us in the first mercy house. We texted back and forth a couple of times a week to encourage each other and to stay up to date on our husbands' progress. Sadly, the clinical trial her husband, Bradley, had been trying had not worked for him, and his cancer was spreading rapidly. One day she texted to let me know they had made the decision to put him on hospice. Bile rose in my throat as I read her words, and I had to fight to keep it down. He had seemed almost fine a few weeks ago when they were in Texas! I dreaded telling Blaine. He was so much more sensitive now than he had ever been before, and any sort of sad news was very, very hard on him. There was no choice though. He needed to know. As expected, he was very sad, and I suspect it scared him. It scared me too. Honestly, it terrified me. Knowing things had changed so quickly for him . . . there are no words. I hate cancer.

Chapter 28

I woke up the next morning to a message on Blaine's Facebook group from our hobby meteorologist friend saying, "Christi and Blaine need prayer." My heart sank as I went on to read the weather report she had attached. A tropical depression was headed toward Houston, and they were predicting fifteen to twenty inches of rain, possibly more than thirty inches in some areas. I made the mistake of clicking the link, and an image of the biggest storm I have ever seen appeared on my phone. I wished I hadn't looked! The report went on to say major catastrophic flooding was coming and everyone in the area must prepare immediately. It was expected to hit the next evening, at exactly the time Blaine had gotten so sick the last two cycles. Considering he had never really recovered from the last one, I was particularly worried this time. Now we were going to have to contend with this storm at the same time.

In Houston the water doesn't drain off the roads when it rains. It just sits there for the longest time. Even with just a quick downpour, standing water stays on the roads, and the traffic goes from annoying to a complete nightmare. I couldn't even begin to imagine what would happen with fifteen to twenty, maybe even thirty-plus, inches of rain! I could stock up on food; we still had the supplies Lydia had brought us for the last storm, and I knew we could move quickly into the big house if the Cottage flooded, but if Blaine needed to go to the ER, I had no idea how I would be able to get him there. Within an hour of seeing the post, it was all over the news. On every channel and everywhere we went, the only thing people were talking about was the storm. It was quickly upgraded and named Hurricane Nicholas. There seemed to be no chance it would miss Houston this time. I couldn't believe we were about to face our second one!

Having spent most of my life in the Midwest with tornados that sprout up seemingly out of the blue, part of me appreciated the amount of warning they were able to give for hurricanes. It was good to have all that time to prepare, but it was also so stressful to just have to wait and wait, knowing what was heading for us. Obviously, there was no choice but to just keep moving forward. It was now day ten, the day Blaine was likely to get really sick. We went to the hospital early that morning to have his labs checked, praying they would somehow be okay and we could ride the storm out in the Cottage.

As we were hoping, his lab results were posted quickly. As we were not hoping, they were already shockingly bad. His white blood cells were down to 0.2; his hemoglobin was down to 6.0, and his platelets were already down to 22. His phosphorus was even down to 1.3, even though they had him taking massive amounts of supplements. I knew under normal circumstances, he would be given a blood transfusion with those numbers, but we were not living in normal circumstances. In addition to all of the COVID consequences everyone talked about, another consequence was that people were not donating blood as they usually did, so there was less available for patients who needed it. The lack of blood for transfusions was a constant issue now at the hospital, and we knew they were having to make very tough decisions on who got it and who didn't. Of course, this was now complicated by the fact the storm was going to hit in a few hours. If Blaine needed a transfusion and we couldn't get there because of the storm, I didn't know what would happen.

Typically, Dr. Baldyga's staff didn't look at the lab results until later in the day, but I think they were worried as well. Veronica called just a few minutes after his results were posted online. "Hello Mrs. Parker." She didn't waste any time with chitchat. "Blaine needs a blood transfusion and some IV phosphorus as soon as possible. We need you to bring him in right now so we can hopefully get you back home before the storm hits." I was so thankful they were on top of this and there was blood for him! I threw my phone charger and his medicine in my bag, and we rushed out the door. As I started the car, I considered running back for my toothbrush and a change of clothes, but I didn't want to waste any time. Plus, we were just going for blood. We would be back in a few hours.

It was already raining by this time, and the wind was blowing pretty hard. The sky had an ominous look I had never seen before. I was so glad we were on our way now and not later when it would be worse. I was pretty worried about the trip back home but managed to mostly put that out of my mind. I could only deal with one problem at a time.

I dropped Blaine off at the ER doors and went to find a parking spot away from the outside edges of the garage, just in case we were still there when the storm got bad. Obviously, everyone else had the same idea, and it took me a long time to find a spot. Finally, I was able to park the car and made a mad dash for the main building, trying not to get completely soaked.

Once again, they already had Blaine in a room and were starting his evaluation by the time I got inside. He felt very tired, but other than that, didn't really seem too sick. He still wasn't talking much, but I was starting to get used to this. The doctor confirmed they were going to give him two units of whole blood and a bag of phosphorus. "If all goes well, you'll be good to head back home in eleven to twelve hours," he said as he hurried out of the room. I did the math in my head. That was going to have us driving home at one a.m., most likely in the height of the hurricane. The roads would be flooded, and it would be dark. I could start to feel the panic swell within me, but I pushed it back down. One problem at a time. I would deal with figuring out how we could safely get back to the Cottage when I had to.

Five minutes later the doctor came back in. "We checked the weather, and it looks like it will not be safe to be outside in twelve hours. We're going to transfer you to a holding floor. That way, when you're done with the transfusions you can just wait there until the storm passes." I let out a huge sigh of relief. Once again, what I had been so worried about never happened. I was thankful the doctor was concerned about our safety even after we left his care. I was also thankful to be out of the ER. I knew on the floor we would have a bigger room with our own bathroom and Blaine would have a more comfortable bed. We would also have a window where I could safely watch the storm go by. It really was the best possible scenario. Surely by tomorrow morning, Blaine would be released, the storm would have passed, and the flooding would have time to go down enough to get back to the Cottage . . . maybe. I was going to hope for the best. Nothing was said about whether or not I could stay with him, and I didn't ask. Surely they wouldn't send me out into the hurricane by myself! My plan was just to act like I had been told to stay and pray no one brought it up.

Thankfully, no one did. Within an hour, they moved Blaine to the holding floor, and I just followed right along. As expected, his new room was much bigger, and it had its own bathroom and a little window. There was no couch for me, but I could last one night in a chair. It would be fine.

The last time he had been in the ER and then was admitted to a floor, the nurses had been wonderful. I was expecting the same experience now, but that's not what we got. While they weren't mean, Blaine clearly was not high on their list of priorities. Maybe they were just overwhelmed with all of the patients they had to care for. Whatever the reason, they seemed annoyed every time they came into his room.

Throughout the day, several times I had to remind them to bring Blaine's medicine. I always waited as long as I possibly could. I knew they were busy, and I did not want to make them think I didn't trust them (even though that was true). I was very aware of a fine line I must not cross. I had to make sure Blaine got the correct treatment, but I also couldn't annoy those in charge of the treatment. We only called them if absolutely necessary, and I just cared for Blaine myself. That was fine with me. I really didn't mind at all, but I was very much looking forward to the change of shift. Surely the night nurses would be more helpful!

Chapter 29

Several hours later, the bags of blood and phosphorus were finally delivered to Blaine's room. Blaine passed the time sleeping. I passed the time staring out the window, waiting for the hurricane, and staring at Blaine, waiting for him to feel better. By the time the blood got there, the night shift had arrived, and his new nurse came to hook the blood to his CVC line.

I was half-asleep but watched with awe as she confidently made all the adjustments to the IV lines, attaching the various tubes to Blaine's CVC lumens, checking all the levels, calibrating the machine to flow at the right speed, pouring the blood into the trash can. My eyes flew open, and I sat up straight to get a good look. She was actually pouring some of the blood out of the IV bag straight into the bathroom trash can! I swallowed slowly, tried not to gag, and forced myself not to think about it. The nurse finally attached the tube from the bag of blood to the CVC line. "There you go," she said curtly as she walked out the door. It appeared the night nurses were not going to be any friendlier than the day shift.

Now there was really nothing to do but sit and wait for the blood to replenish Blaine's body and hopefully give him more energy. I was sitting next to him scrolling through my phone, and he was just lying in the bed when all of a sudden alarms started going off. I quickly looked at the monitor and saw that his oxygen saturation had dropped dangerously. I looked over at Blaine. He was looking back at me completely perplexed but breathing just fine. "Are you feeling okay? Are you getting in enough air?"

"I'm fine."

We waited a minute or two, but no one came, so we pushed the call button for the nurse. Someone different came in to check on him. He confirmed Blaine was indeed breathing just fine, reset the monitor, and left. A few minutes later, it happened again. "Are you sure you don't feel short of breath?"

"I'm fine."

I pushed the call button again, and the nurse came back, confirmed Blaine was okay, reset the monitor, and left again. For no apparent reason whatsoever, the alarm just kept going off, indicating Blaine was not getting enough oxygen. Finally, the nurse said, "You know, we can just turn this off if you want."

I was getting pretty annoyed at the constant interruption, but I wasn't sure it was a good idea just to turn it off. What if he actually did start to have trouble breathing or had another problem? "Don't you need to know if something's wrong?"

"Oh! We get an alarm at the nurse's desk. We'll be notified there and will come to check on him, but you won't have to listen to the noise."

"You're sure someone is sitting there monitoring it?"

"Oh, of course. Someone is there at all times. If anything is wrong, we'll come."

This made me a tiny bit uncomfortable, but the noise really was disturbing, and I felt confident the staff would keep him safe, so I agreed. He made the adjustment to the monitoring system and left again.

A little while later, Blaine needed to use the restroom. One arm was attached to the IV pole with the bags of blood, phosphorus, and fluid. On his other side, the monitor was attached to his finger. There was no way for him to get out of the bed. The obvious answer was to call the nurse so she could unhook him, but there was no time for that. He almost never had any significant warning now before he urgently needed a restroom. There was certainly no time to wait for a nurse, so in typical Blaine fashion, he ripped the monitor right off his finger and climbed out of the bed. I grabbed the IV pole and hurried along behind him. While we couldn't hear any noise, one look at the monitor confirmed it was going crazy. I expected the nurse to come flying in at any second to make sure he was okay.

She didn't. Blaine finished up in the restroom and got back into the bed. We waited. No one came. His monitor was flashing like it was about to blow up. No one came. After twenty minutes, my patience was gone. I punched the call button so hard it hurt my finger. A little while later, one of the techs came in and asked if she could help us. I couldn't even answer her. I just pointed to the flashing monitor. "Oh! Are you feeling all right Mr. Parker?"

"Yeah."

She reset the monitor as I explained that he had unhooked it twenty minutes ago. I paused and took a deep, steadying breath, determined not to lose my cool. "Doesn't it seem like maybe someone should have come to check on him?"

"Umm. . . Let me get the nurse."

A few minutes later the top person on the floor during the night came in to explain what happened. "We were away from the desk and did not notice his alarm going off."

"I thought someone was monitoring it."

"Oh! Of course there's someone monitoring it!"

"You just said no one noticed it."

"There's an office in another building where people monitor the alarms."

This seemed strange to me, but I let it go. "Well, they don't seem to be doing a very good job. He took it off twenty minutes ago and no one was sent to check on him."

"That's because they could tell he had just taken it off. If there were an emergency, they would have notified us."

"And what would happen if there were an emergency, and he didn't have the monitor on?"

"Well, there wasn't, was there? He seems fine."

Obviously, this was going nowhere. I let it go. While I completely did not mind taking care of Blaine's basic needs, and in fact really preferred that to letting the nurses care for him, I desperately did need to feel that someone was there if an emergency arose, that I could relax and trust the professionals to take care of all of his medical issues. Instead, it seemed I had to be on extra-high alert with them. I needed to make sure they were bringing him the right medicines at the right times, and now I even had to make sure they were paying attention to his monitor in case something serious went wrong. Blaine was speaking less and less. He seemed to be getting sicker. I did not know why, and I did not have any sense the nurses were paying attention at all.

He went back to sleep while I stared obsessively at his vital signs on the monitor. I noticed his heart rate stayed at a pretty regular sixty to seventy beats per minute when he was lying down, but when he sat up, it would be a little higher. I understand the heart beats a little faster when a person moves around, but Blaine's seemed to be jumping higher than I would have expected. That seemed odd to me, but it wasn't too drastic of a jump, so I wasn't really worried.

I alternated between sitting in the chair right next to Blaine's bed and the chair next to the window, watching for the hurricane. I quickly discovered that I had vastly overestimated how comfortable that chair would be. It was going to be a long night. On a positive note, nothing scary seemed to be happening outside. It was raining, and the wind was blowing a bit, but that was it. Every time I checked the weather, the storm's anticipated arrival had been pushed a little further back. It was maddening to just sit and wait for it to hit.

I did my best to sleep, but it was impossible to find a comfortable position, and just when I might start to doze off, Blaine would need me to jump up to help him to the restroom. It seemed that every time he got up, his heart rate was shooting higher and higher. I was starting to get more and more concerned. When it started hitting 150 consistently every time he sat up, I was really worried. I finally broke down and asked someone to come check on him.

A nurse came in fairly quickly, and I described what was happening. "Oh, that's totally normal, nothing to worry about," she said.

"It's normal to have that big of a jump?"

"Of course! Everyone's heart rate jumps when they are active."

This didn't seem right to me, but she was a highly-trained medical professional, and I was not. Plus, it was 4 a.m., and I had been awake for approximately twenty-two hours at that point. Surely, she must know what she was talking about.

A little while later I got an email notifying me that Blaine's latest lab results had been posted. I obsessed over his lab results as much as I did his vital signs. The labs weren't good. His hemoglobin was up a bit, thanks to the blood transfusion, but his platelets were down to 14. Most concerning though, his white count was down to 0.1! How is it even possible to have a white count of 0.1? He had absolutely no defense against any pathogen that might come his way. All I could think about was our friend, Kathy, who had died from a mouth sore because her body didn't have the resources to fight the infection. I was terrified to even breathe in his direction. The staff had told me earlier that we could take our masks off when we were alone in the room, but now I put mine back on and scooted away from him. I wasn't taking any chances!

Chapter 30

A few hours later, the physician assigned to the holding floor came to check on Blaine. He explained that his lab counts still were not where they needed to be in order for him to be discharged, but he was hoping they would rebound soon. He asked Blaine how he was feeling. Blaine didn't answer. He just stared at him. I never knew what my role was in times like this. I didn't want him to feel I was mothering him, but I needed the doctor to have all the information. It was always an uncomfortable situation for me. I'm sure I irritated Blaine occasionally when I answered for him, but sometimes there was no choice.

This was one of those times. Blaine just kept staring at the doctor. He had been talking less and less, but this was the first time someone asked him a direct question and he just didn't answer. Finally, I spoke up. "He's not complaining of anything specific, but he really doesn't seem to feel good. He's sleeping most of the time and not talking very much at all, and for some reason, every time he sits up, his heart rate shoots up to 150."

"His heart rate is jumping when he sits up?" Suddenly the doctor seemed much more concerned than he had a few seconds ago.

"Yes, when he's lying still the monitor shows it's between 60 and 70, but as soon as he sits up, it jumps to around 150 or so. The nurse told me it was fine."

The doctor told his assistant to order some more lab tests and then turned back to me. "That is not fine at all. It's a sign his body may be fighting a serious infection. His white count is only 0.1, so if he has any sort of an infection, this is very concerning. We'll have them run some more tests, and we'll let you know what they show. We're also going to go ahead and order a platelet transfusion for him. Typically, we don't transfuse platelets until they drop below 10 now, but his are clearly heading in the wrong direction, and I want to make sure he gets them."

I thanked them, and they left to see their next patient. Very soon after, a lab tech came in to take some more blood for the new tests, and in a surprisingly short amount of time after that, his bag of platelets for the transfusion arrived. I breathed out a sigh of relief, thankful things were finally happening quickly.

The day nurse also came in during this time. I was so glad she was not the same one from the day before. I could tell right away that Toula was wonderful. She came to introduce herself and to check on Blaine. She was warm and friendly, and even more importantly, she seemed to know what she was doing. His meds were always on time (and accurate); she answered all of my questions, and she just generally took care of him in a way that allowed me to relax a little. I loved Toula!

She wrapped up her assessment of Blaine and looked me in the eyes. "How are *you* doing, Christi?"

My initial instinct was to tell her I was fine but decided I should be honest. "I think I might be starving to death."

"Oh, honey! You need to eat!"

"I'm pretty sure I'm not supposed to be here. I don't want to risk being caught."

"I think it will be okay. Just act like everything is fine, and most likely no one will question you. Go! Go! I'll keep a close eye on your hubby."

I was getting pretty good at acting like I knew what I was doing, and no one seemed to even notice me. As I stepped off the elevator onto Blaine's floor with my food, I almost ran into the physician's assistant who had been with the doctor that morning. "Oh! Mrs. Parker, I was just looking for you!" She paused. This couldn't be good. "I'm afraid I have some not great news. Your husband's procalcitonin level came back very elevated. This indicates a high likelihood of sepsis. We're going to start him on IV antibiotics and admit him to the regular floor."

I thanked her and headed back to Blaine's room to Google procalcitonin levels and eat my lunch/dinner/breakfast. Toula came in soon to start his antibiotics and explained they would get him moved to the regular floor as soon as a bed was available. Unfortunately, the hospital was full and there was no way of knowing when that might be. We spent the day waiting. Blaine slept most of the day. I sat most of the day. I tried to read books on my phone, but it was hard to concentrate. Blaine barely spoke the whole day. The hours crept by. They brought another bag of blood and eventually another bag of IV antibiotics.

As it became apparent we would be spending another night on the holding floor, I tried to convince Toula to stay for the night shift. She was wonderful, but she had her limits! She laughed at my attempts and told us all about her kids and husband waiting for her at home. I finally agreed she should probably go, but I was quite worried about getting through another night with the same staff as before.

A little while later, Toula came in to check on Blaine one last time and to tell us goodbye. I thanked her profusely for everything, and she started to leave. She hesitated as she was opening the door and then turned back around. She seemed sort of uncomfortable, but finally said, "I sense that you two are Christians. Am I right?"

My eyes widened. "Yes, we are!" While we were determined to be a light for Christ at this hospital, the last twenty-four hours we had just been trying to survive. I don't think we did anything un-Christlike, but we also hadn't been going out of our way to talk to anyone about God.

"I knew it!" she exclaimed. "God wants me to tell you that He loves you and He's pleased with you. He is taking care of you." I sat frozen in my chair, completely unable to make a sound. All of a sudden, my husband, who had barely spoken five words all day, started this long speech about how God was also pleased with her, that she had a very important ministry at the hospital and was exactly where God wanted her to be. I just stared at him with my mouth hanging open. I wasn't shocked at what he said, but I was amazed that he was speaking that much at all!

Toula was also amazed. She went on to tell us all about how she had left her home country to minister in America and how she felt it was her mission to share God's love with the patients and their families in this hospital. She asked if she could pray for Blaine and then proceeded to give the most Spirit-filled prayer I have ever heard. She prayed for his complete healing and for our girls at home, our finances, the tiny details involved in maintaining our lives while fighting cancer, and for our peace and spiritual strength. At some point she lapsed into her native language, but somehow we still had a good idea of what she was saying. I sensed God's presence in the room in a way I had never experienced before. I prayed for her as well, and then she said goodbye and finally went home to her family. I thought we would surely see her again, but we never did. I was so grateful that she had been assigned to Blaine that day. Based on her prayer, I was sure he must have been cured and the worst of all of this mess was behind us!

Chapter 31

Since that day's crew had been so much better than the ones from the day before, I was cautiously optimistic there would be new night staff also. Thankfully, I was right! James, the night nurse, walked in a little while after Toula left to introduce himself. Time would tell, but my first impression was that he seemed completely together. I started to hope maybe that night wouldn't be as bad.

Sometime later, Blaine needed to use the restroom, so he unhooked his monitor, and I helped with the IV pole. I had barely gotten the door closed when James came rushing into the room asking if he was okay. "Oh, he's fine," I replied. "He just unhooked the monitor so he could use the restroom."

"Okay, good! I saw the alarm go off at the desk and was worried something had happened."

Ugly thoughts about the last night's nurses bombarded my mind, but I kept them to myself.

Blaine got into the bed, put the monitor on his finger, and quickly went back to sleep. I tried unsuccessfully to get comfortable in the chair. By this point, I had been awake for around forty hours, and I could barely hold my eyes open. Eventually sleep won, and I dozed off.

"Christi!" My eyes flew open, and I tried to make sense of where I was. Blaine was standing up trying to get himself to the restroom and very irritated I wasn't helping. He couldn't get there by himself, and he really had to move quickly to prevent an embarrassing accident. I knew he had no idea how tired I was. Somehow my body went into action before my brain even registered what was happening. By the time I woke up, I was already halfway across the room. I managed to grab the pole and get him to the restroom just in time.

This little scenario repeated itself many, many times over the next week. I somehow learned to sleep without really sleeping. I never knew when he would need something, and I had to be ready.

In addition to the nighttime emergency restroom trips, as everyone knows, the night staff at hospitals must check patient's vital signs, take blood, and do other random things during the night. Hospitals are definitely not the place to get rest! At some point in the night, a tech came in to do her scheduled assessment. I was able to see Blaine's blood pressure and pulse on the monitor, but I always had to ask about his temperature. "How's everything look?" I asked as she finished up.

"His temperature is 102.3."

At that point, I'm sure *my* blood pressure and pulse shot up. How could he have a fever? He had gotten two bags of strong IV antibiotics!

"I'll get James," she said as she hurried out of the room.

Soon James rushed back in. As he was making sure there were no other problems, he told me, "I've already called the doctor and he's already ordered a different antibiotic. It will be ready in just a few minutes." I thanked him and hugged my knees to my chest, trying to keep myself from panicking. How could he possibly have a fever after two bags of antibiotics? I knew that was a very bad sign. If he had an infection the antibiotics weren't effective against . . .

The tech brought in the new bag of antibiotics a few minutes later, and James got it going. He continued to keep very close tabs on Blaine all through the night. I really did trust his ability and determination to keep Blaine as safe as possible, but sleep was out of the question at this point. I spent the rest of the night alternating between begging God to heal him and just staring at him numbly. Time dragged so slowly. A few hours after

James started the new antibiotic, Blaine's fever finally went down to 100.7, still not great, but definitely better.

Around 7:00 the next morning, a bed finally opened up in the main part of the hospital. I tried really hard not to think about why a bed would suddenly be available at seven in the morning. James took us upstairs and introduced us to the floor nurses. He gave them all of Blaine's important information, and then it was time for him to go. My voice caught as I told him goodbye. I felt like I was losing a friend when he walked out the door, and I was terrified of being in charge of Blaine's care again. I had learned that it was not safe to assume the nurses would do a good job.

Chapter 32

Not long after we arrived on the floor, Dr. Linus and his assistant stopped in to introduce themselves and see how Blaine was doing. All of the sarcoma doctors take one-week shifts being in charge of the hospital patients, and we happened to be there during Dr. Linus' shift. He asked Blaine how he was feeling, and as usual, he told him he was feeling okay. Dr. Linus took a quick look at Lumpy and then inside Blaine's mouth. He confirmed Blaine was starting to have some mucositis and a couple of mouth sores.

He sat in a chair to chat. He confirmed Blaine and I knew chemotherapy works by attacking rapidly dividing cells and explained that in addition to tumor cells, the epithelial cells that line the gastrointestinal tract also divide rapidly so the chemotherapy attacks those as well. Sometimes this causes mucositis, which is increased mucus and thicker saliva, and can leave the mucosal tissue open to ulceration and infection. "We'll watch those sores closely. Make sure to keep up on your swish and spit/swish and swallow medicines. Those should help." We assured him we would, and he went on.

"We are still waiting on a few tests, but so far everything has come back negative for any specific infection. We think you are just suffering from neutropenic sepsis." He went on to explain that half of the patients on Blaine's specific chemo regimen were hospitalized with neutropenic sepsis every cycle. He looked me in the eyes. "We will be watching him very closely, but he should make a full recovery."

Somehow, I took this to mean there wasn't any real infection, and he wasn't in any real danger at the moment. Unfortunately, I later Googled neutropenic sepsis and was shocked to learn that neutropenic sepsis is considered to be an emergency situation and is a major cause of death in people with neutropenia.

Note to self: *DON'T GOOGLE!*

Even when I believed the neutropenic sepsis wasn't as bad as I later learned it to be, it seemed obvious the chemo needed to stop. Dr. Linus seemed very logical to me, so I broached the subject with him. "Have you read much of Blaine's history?"

"Yes, I've seen his file."

"So you know the tumor has had a fantastic response to the chemotherapy, that it is much smaller now than when he started?"

"Yes, I saw that. That's really impressive."

"Don't you think if the chemo was so effective against the formed mass of sarcoma cells, if there happened to be any random microscopic cells floating around his body, they would have been completely obliterated by now?"

"That is what we are hoping for."

"Then doesn't it seem a little crazy to keep risking his life with the chemo when surely those cells are gone?"

Dr. Linus sighed. "That is something that you will need to discuss with Dr. Baldyga, but I can tell you that years of research has proven that six cycles of chemotherapy should be the standard treatment plan."

Now it was my turn to sigh. This was really not the response I was hoping for. I hated to remind Blaine about Kathy, but I needed Dr. Linus to know that I knew how serious this white count issue was. Blaine, of course, already knew about Kathy, and I wasn't totally sure how much he was paying attention to our conversation anyway, so I plunged in. "A few years ago, we had a good friend receiving chemotherapy. One night, she needed to stay in the hospital to receive IV fluids because she had gotten dehydrated. She also happened to have a mouth sore and a depressed white count. Her husband told her goodnight and drove twenty minutes to his house, fully expecting to pick her up in the morning. The infection from the mouth sore spread. She was in a coma by the time he got home, even though she had seemed fine when he left," I paused and swallowed hard. I was trying so hard to keep my voice from cracking. "And then she died."

Dr. Linus sat silently for a moment. "I am so sorry about your friend." He paused and then looked straight at me with actual tears in his eyes. "I promise we will do absolutely everything possible to keep Blaine safe." I felt my fear ease just a bit. I've never known a doctor who seemed as invested in a patient, and I instantly trusted him.

We chatted for a few more minutes and then Dr. Linus and his assistant left to see their other patients, promising to let us know what the remaining labs showed.

The rest of the day passed fairly uneventfully. There was a couch in the room with a little blanket, and I dozed off and on. At some point I thought to ask the nurse if they happened to have any extra toothbrushes, and when she brought me one with a little tube of toothpaste, it felt like the greatest gift I had ever received! It is amazing what having clean teeth can do for your outlook on life! I vowed never, ever to take Blaine to the ER again without having a toothbrush with me—even if there was a hurricane coming.

Blaine slept most of the day. He was talking less and less and ignoring people more and more. Frequently when I, or someone else, asked him a question, he just didn't respond at all. I started to wonder sometimes if he was even aware anyone was in the room with him. His fever continued to spike through the day, going as high as 102.9. Dr. Linus told me his white count was so low, it might take a few days for the antibiotics to start working. Thankfully, the nurses on the floor were great, and they kept a very close eye on him.

Even though it felt as if Blaine and I were dealing with a hurricane inside, the one outside had just disappeared. At one point that evening, the mayor of Houston appeared on the news and said, "Houston was blessed. I'm not going to say we were lucky. God blessed Houston in protecting us from Nicholas." I just shook my head. It didn't seem possible that we had been threatened with not one, but two full-blown hurricanes and God had totally protected us from both!

Although time seemed to be standing still, I could tell by the clock it was getting closer and closer to 8 p.m., the time visiting hours were over and I assumed I would be booted out of the hospital. Nothing had been said about what time I needed to leave. I planned to act like I was fine to stay and hope no one noticed me, but the anticipation of being kicked out any minute was making me feel even more anxious, so I finally broke down and asked the nurse if I needed to go.

"Oh no! You're on the approved list. You can stay as long as necessary!"

My heart jumped in my throat, first with joy, but then with fear. I knew the only way I would be on the list is if Blaine had been classified as either mentally incapacitated or near death. Either was terrifying, so I refused to think about it. I decided to push it just a little. "Am I allowed to leave the room?"

"Of course! You can't go outside the building and then come back in, but you're free to roam around inside the hospital as much as you want."

I called Lydia to let her know I was going to be staying at the hospital, and she offered to bring us some clean clothes. By this point, we had been wearing the same clothes for three days, and the idea of being able to put on something clean made me feel like the luckiest woman alive. Lydia would have to deal with the traffic around the hospital and park her truck so she could meet me inside the doors, but she didn't even hesitate. I ran down to meet her an hour later and felt the tension in my body relax when I saw her familiar face. In addition to the clothes, she also brought a big bag of snacks and drinks and a few books. This was not her first rodeo. She knew what we would need more than I did.

I hugged her and rushed back to the room to be with Blaine. He was sleeping, and I don't think he even knew I was gone. I settled down on the little couch and tried to rest. Blaine did need help several times through the night, and his fever continued to rise and fall, but all things considered, it was much more peaceful than the night before. I thought surely his white count would start to bounce back tomorrow and the worst was behind us.

Chapter 33

In the early morning hours, way before the sun was up, a tech came in to take blood from Blaine's CVC. Blaine barely seemed to notice he was there. I was so anxious to see what his levels were that I didn't even care he had ruined some actual sleeping time for me. The tech got what he needed, and I tried to get a little more rest. Before long, one of the nurse's aides came in to check his vitals. I gave up sleeping and sat up so I could ask what his temperature was.

"Good morning," I said. "How is your day going so far?"

"Pretty good! How about yours? Were you able to get any sleep?"

"Enough," I lied.

"Oh! Your husband's name is Blaine! One of the main characters in my favorite movie was named Blaine! Have you ever seen *Pretty in Pink*?"

"Yes! That is one of my favorite movies too! I always thought Blaine was the best name ever!"

"Me too!" she gushed. Weirdly enough, she is the only other person I have ever come across who had this opinion. Clearly, it's the best name ever.

"What's his temperature?"

"102." She sighed. "It's going to be okay. The antibiotics just need time to work. I'll be back in a little while to check on him."

She walked out of the room, and I picked up my phone to see what was happening in the real world. A few minutes later she came back. She was hiding something under her sweater.

"Here, I was able to snag a blanket for you. I thought you might like it."

I sucked in my breath in surprise and tried my best not to squeal. I took it from her and hugged it tight. It was a real, actual, warm blanket! I don't know why those were such a rarity, but in all the time I had spent in that hospital over the last several weeks, I had never been offered an actual blanket. I vowed to guard it with my life!

A little while later Dr. Linus's assistant, Catalina, and a student walked into the room. Every morning, the assistants made rounds checking on patients and then briefed the physician about their condition before they came in a while later. "How are you feeling today, Mr. Parker?" she asked with a smile.

He barely even looked at her. Finally, I spoke up. "He's not talking much, but I'm pretty sure he's not feeling good at all."

She looked at him sympathetically. "I'm so sorry, Mr. Parker. Once your counts start to come back up, I know you'll feel better."

"When do you expect that to be?" I asked.

"There's no way to tell. Everyone responds to chemotherapy differently. We just have to wait and see." We had been told this many times before, and it made Blaine crazy.

All of a sudden, he came to life. He actually yelled at Catalina. "This is such a crock! You people can do whatever you want to us and have no responsibility whatsoever. 'Everyone responds differently,'" he mocked. "That means nothing. You have no idea what's going to happen after you put that stuff in us."

He kept going, but I stopped listening. My ribs suddenly seemed too tight for my body as I tried to remember to breathe and stared helplessly at the scene unfolding. I felt so bad. I felt bad for Blaine because I knew he must feel completely awful to actually be yelling at this poor woman. He never acted like that. I felt bad for Catalina who had no choice but to stand there and take it. I felt bad for myself because everything about the situation was awful.

At some point Catalina glanced over at me, and I mouthed the words, "I am so sorry." She nodded her head a little. I'm sure this was not the first time she had been yelled at by a patient, but I still agonized for her. Finally, Blaine stopped and relaxed back into his pillow. "Mr. Parker, I know it's frustrating, and I am sorry you are feeling bad. I will let Dr. Linus know, and we will do everything we can to make you as comfortable as possible." Blaine ignored her. She and the student turned to leave, and I gave them a little apologetic smile. It was the only thing I could do.

When Dr. Linus came in an hour or so later, he looked in Blaine's mouth and throat and discovered they were now completely full of sores. He let us know his labs showed his white count was still at 0.1 and his platelets were down to 5. He had ordered a bag of platelets to be transfused, but sadly informed us that until Blaine's body was able to make more white cells, there was really nothing more they could do about the sores. He was on multiple strong IV antibiotics, but it really all hinged on Blaine's own white cells. Until those started to come back, nothing would get better.

On his way out the door to see his next patient, Dr. Linus paused and rested his hand on my shoulder. The warmth from his fingers spread through me, and I felt less alone. Friends and family constantly sent texts or Facebook messages letting me know they were thinking of us, but I was really all alone with this. Dr. Linus's compassion made me stronger. Nothing had changed about our situation, but in that moment, it suddenly seemed more manageable.

Blaine promptly went back to sleep, and I decided to try to do the same. I snuggled down under my new piece of heaven and felt my tension ease as the soft fabric enveloped me. In addition to feeling warmer than I had in days, having my body wrapped up somehow made me feel safer as well, and I quickly dozed off.

Prior to receiving any sort of transfusion, patients are given Benadryl and Tylenol. Some days the Benadryl had more of an effect on Blaine than others. Today it knocked him out cold. When the nurse came back in to start the platelets, I asked if she thought it would be a good time for me to take a shower.

"I think that's a great idea! We'll keep an eye on him, but my guess is he'll sleep right through."

I grabbed my clean clothes and hurried into the bathroom. I was afraid Blaine would wake up and think he was alone, so I showered in record time, but it was still the greatest thing ever. I now had a clean body, clean clothes, and a blanket. I felt like a new woman!

When I rushed back into the room, Blaine was still completely asleep. I settled down on the couch for a long day of waiting. I waited for his white count to rise. I waited for his temperature to drop. I waited for him to wake up and talk to me like normal. There was absolutely nothing I could do about any of those things. I had zero control. All I could do was wait.

Actually, there was something I did besides wait; I caught mucus. Multiple times an hour, Blaine would grab the little pink, kidney-shaped emesis basin and try to spit. I would hold the dish for him while he worked to expel a huge mass of mucus from his mouth. It was long and thick and stringy. To get it all, he had to reach into his mouth and pull it out with his fingers. Sometimes it was so long he actually seemed to be pulling it up from his stomach. Often there would be big chunks of skin and/or blood. I would just stand there holding the basin, praying he wouldn't choke, praying I wouldn't vomit. When he finished, I washed it out in the sink. I acted cool, like it was no big deal, but . . . it was.

That afternoon I was scrolling aimlessly through my phone while Blaine was sleeping. All of a sudden, he sucked in his breath and grabbed his abdomen. I rushed over to his bed, my heart racing as I imagined all the horrible things that could be causing the pain. "What's wrong?"

He kept his eyes closed tight, his face in a deep grimace, and pointed to his stomach. "It hurts?" I asked. He nodded. Then as quickly as the pain had come, it seemed to vanish. Blaine relaxed and went back to sleep. I pushed the button to call the nurse. She came quickly and I told her what had happened. He was sleeping again and seemed fine, so she advised we just continue to keep an eye on him.

He slept most of the rest of the day. He had a few more of those random pains, but none of them lasted long. I spent the day scrolling through Facebook, reading some books, staring at Blaine, and staring out the window. There was a little TV by my couch, but I didn't want to disturb Blaine, so I didn't watch it. I texted with the girls and a few other family members and friends. It was a long day.

That evening, just as I decided I would try to go to sleep, a tech came in to check Blaine's temperature. I waited patiently for the number, mentally preparing myself for bad news. I was stunned when she turned around beaming and proclaimed, "*No fever*!"

"What? Really?" I thought maybe I had heard wrong. My heart seemed to jump into my throat, and my skin tingled. I couldn't wipe the smile off my face. This was the first good news in days!

"It's actually 98.7!" She was excited too. I loved that most of the staff seemed to genuinely care about how he was doing! She wrapped up her tasks and left so we could get some sleep. I snuggled down under my new blanket and thanked God over and over. Dr. Linus had warned me his fever would probably bounce around until his white blood cells came back, and I knew it was likely to go back up, but for this particular moment, I was just going to cling to the idea that it would stay down, that the worst was over. The blanket and the belief that Blaine was recovering were powerful sedatives, and although I did need to be up with him several times through the night, I rested better than I had since we arrived at the hospital, which was good. I was going to need it.

Chapter 34

I awoke the next morning to an unfamiliar noise. The phone by the bed was ringing. I ran to answer it before it disturbed Blaine. "Hello?"

"Mrs. Parker?"

"Yes."

"Hello! My name is Susan, and I am a nutritionist here at the hospital. How are you today?"

"I'm fine. How are you?" I said a little warily.

"I'm good, but we're worried about your husband. We've been monitoring his weight, and it is dropping significantly. What has he been eating?"

"Honestly? Not much. I can get him to sip on a Boost now and then, but basically, he just does not want to swallow anything. He has terrible sores. He can't stand anything that is too hot or too cold and everything tastes salty to him."

"You have to get him to eat. At the absolute minimum, he must get at least three cans of Boost down every day. If he cannot do that, we're going to have to put in a feeding tube."

My heart sank. In the back of my mind, I knew this was a possibility, but I somehow wasn't expecting it this soon. I assured her I would do everything I could to get him to eat. She offered suggestions for foods he might like, all of which I knew he would refuse because they were too cold. She explained that his life was in jeopardy if he couldn't take in enough calories. Of course I knew that, but hearing the words spoken aloud felt like a hard slap. I thanked her and hung up the phone.

Blaine was staring at me. "That was the nutritionist. Here, would you like a sip of Boost?" I tried to hand him the container, but he shook his head. I sighed. "Honey, they are very concerned about your weight. I need you to drink this." He shook his head again. "They're going to put in a feeding tube if you won't eat." He shook his head again.

I didn't know what to do. When Blaine makes up his mind about something, there's nothing anyone can do to change it. The idea of him slowly starving to death terrified me. I knew they would put in a feeding tube before it got that far, but for some reason, that scared me too. Tears started running down my cheeks. During this whole ordeal, I had managed not to cry in front of him, but now I was powerless to hold it back. "Honey, after all you've been through, you can't let yourself die because you won't eat. I know it's hard, but you have to fight. They call it 'fighting cancer.' Maybe this is what they mean. You can't let it win. I need you to fight. I *need* you to eat." I hung my head and just cried. I was so scared, but I knew there was nothing I could do.

"Okay," he whispered.

My head shot back up. "Did you say okay?"

He nodded his head, and I held the container of Boost with the straw up to his lips. He took a sip. I was so relieved! He took another sip, and then I could tell he was done.

"She said you need to be drinking three of these a day at the absolute minimum."

"Okay."

I handed the container back to him. He took it and slowly drank the whole thing. I don't think I have ever loved him more than at that moment. I knew he felt awful, but he was going to fight for me! That one container was all he managed to get down that day, and it would be a while before he drank three in one day, but somehow his weight stopped falling, and there was no more talk of the feeding tube.

Dr. Linus came in a little while later. He was thrilled Blaine had managed to drink a whole container of Boost and reiterated that he needed to be drinking at least three a day. He then gave us the unfortunate news that Blaine's white count was still at 0.1. I couldn't believe it wasn't rising at all! His other lab values remained right on the edge of necessitating yet another blood transfusion. They were going to hold off for the moment because there simply wasn't enough available for nonemergency situations, but they would monitor him closely.

Although there didn't seem to be a connection with Blaine swallowing the Boost, his random stomach pains continued. They became more frequent and were even more painful than the day before. He had a couple while Dr. Linus was in the room, and he felt sure that Blaine had developed mouth sores all the way down to his stomach. He ordered IV morphine in hopes that would assuage the pain, but it didn't seem to even touch it. It was a long, awful day.

The only positive point came that afternoon when I checked my email. There was a message from the hospital asking me to donate blood since Blaine was needing so much. I had tried to donate as soon as I learned their supply was low but was told because of COVID, they were only accepting donations from employees. I was glad to learn that information was wrong and quickly let them know I would be happy to help. They wrote back with instructions on where to go, and I told Blaine what was happening so he would know where I was if he woke up and I was gone.

A little while later, he did finally seem to fall into a deep sleep, so I slipped out quietly and found the room where they took the blood donations. Other than to meet Lydia to grab our clothes, I hadn't been outside of Blaine's room in days. It was a little disorienting, but I'm sure it was good for me. I had never given blood before, but the process was quick and easy, and I was so happy I was able to contribute a little bit back. When they were finished, they gave me a snack and I zipped back up to Blaine's room. I'm not sure he ever knew I had left. Just being out of the room for a bit seemed to give me new energy,[10] and knowing I had helped with the blood supply gave me peace that I wouldn't worry so much the next time Blaine needed a transfusion. Unfortunately, that time would come soon.

Chapter 35

Early the next morning, Dr. Linus walked in grinning from ear to ear. "Mr. Parker! Your white count has doubled!"

I sat up groggily. I had actually been sleeping and couldn't quite process what he meant. "What did you say?"

"I said it's doubled! His white count has *doubled*!"

Now I was awake! Doubled? That was incredible! Slowly though, I realized what he meant. "You mean it's 0.2."

"Well, yes, but technically that's double what it's been!"

I laughed. Zero-point-two was still frighteningly awful, but I loved Dr. Linus's attitude!

"Unfortunately, while your white count finally seems to be moving in the right direction, your hemoglobin is down to 6.2 and your platelets are down to 3." I couldn't even comprehend someone having a platelet level of 3! I remembered the day I was so worried when they dropped to 9. Having a platelet count of 3 was crazy. I knew he could bleed to death quickly if he even just bumped something. "I've ordered two units of whole blood and a bag of platelets. They should be here soon. How's your pain today?"

No response from Blaine. We all stared at him for a moment, and then I gave up and answered, "I think it's pretty bad."

Dr. Linus' smile vanished. "Okay, we'll get some more morphine going too." He chatted for a few more minutes and then left to see his other patients.

Soon the nurse brought in the morphine, and a little while later, the bag of platelets and one bag of blood. "I know Dr. Linus ordered two bags, but the blood department said there simply isn't enough on hand. We'll give him this, and hopefully it will help," she said as she hooked the bags to Blaine's CVC line.

I was expecting this day to come, but it was so unsettling when it actually did. I suspect there were times when Blaine would have been given a transfusion if there had been plenty of blood available, but he wasn't. They needed to save what they had for more critical patients. They had always managed to have it, though, when he absolutely needed it, and the fact they didn't have enough now was terrifying.

We spent the afternoon watching the Alabama football team beat the Florida Gators while lifesaving blood slowly dripped into Blaine's body. It was such an odd sensation to be doing such a normal autumn Saturday afternoon activity in such a completely different environment, but it was a pretty good day. The morphine somehow helped more than it had the day before, and Blaine was much more interactive than he had been for the last several days. Maybe that was more an effect of Alabama football than the morphine, but either way, it made me happy. Later in the evening, the blood department even decided they could spare another unit, so Blaine ended up getting what he needed after all. Things were definitely looking up!

The next morning, though, things were not so cheery. All of his lab numbers looked better than they had for the last eight days, but Blaine felt worse. He was ignoring people completely. A nurse would walk in and ask him a question, and he would act like he didn't even know anyone was there. Sometimes I would say something, and he would give no indication he was aware I was even in the room. He had been doing this intermittently for the last several days, but today it was consistent. I was never quite sure if he just did not feel like responding, or if he truly was unaware we were there. Either way, it scared me.

Dr. Baldyga had warned us in the beginning about the neurological compromise. She had promised it wouldn't be permanent, but what if she was wrong? Over and over we had been told, "Everyone responds to chemotherapy differently." What if he didn't come out of this? I tried to think logically. I knew none of his symptoms were a shock to the doctors, so it was likely he would return mentally, like all the other patients. It was easy to say that, but trusting it was so hard! While I watched him seem to slip further and further away from me, I had to remind myself over and over that it would not be permanent, that the day was coming when this would all be behind us and he would be back to normal.

Blaine's regression was particularly concerning because I needed to fly home the next day. At that point, the girls had not seen a parent for five weeks. If I didn't go home during this little window before the next chemo cycle was scheduled to start, it would be at least three more weeks before I could leave, and that was if there were no complications, which seemed unlikely. It just wasn't right to leave them without any parents for that long! I discussed it with Dr. Linus before I booked the flight, and he had said he thought it would be fine. I asked him again that morning, and he still said he thought it was fine, although he said it a little more slowly, as if he didn't love the idea. I felt like the worst wife in the world. I couldn't believe I was going to leave Blaine, but I couldn't completely abandon our children. Blaine's father and stepmother were making the drive from Missouri that day so they could take care of Blaine while I was at home. They were going to spend the night in the Cottage while I spent one more night in the hospital.

My last day at the hospital passed fairly uneventfully, and soon it was time for bed. I did not sleep at all. I jumped every time Blaine stirred the slightest bit. If he was awake, I needed to pour as much love into him as I possibly could. Plus, if I happened to doze off a little, some random thing would pop into my head that I needed to remember to tell the nurses.

I was confident they would do an excellent job taking care of the big things, but there were a million little things he needed during the day, and especially during the night, they didn't necessarily know about. For instance, every few hours they would bring his pills in a little cup and set them on the table that went over his bed, assuming he would take them. They did not know how much work it was to get him to actually swallow them all. He would take one at a time and then wait what seemed like an eternity to take the next one. Some days it felt like my main responsibility was to remind him to take his pills over and over and over again. Who was going to do that if I wasn't there?

I also realized I needed to tell them not to say too many words to him at once. While frequently he would seem to ignore people, sometimes he would get upset when someone talked to him. I had finally figured out he was having trouble processing more than one sentence at a time and had learned to translate important information to him in small bits. It occurred to me in the middle of the night that I had to be sure to tell them this before I left, but would they remember? Maybe I shouldn't go.

But how much damage had already been done to my relationship with the girls by being gone for five weeks? I couldn't make it eight, or most likely even more. I had to go.

But my first responsibility was to my husband. I had to stay.

But I was a mother too. I had to go.

I probably changed my mind twenty times during the night about whether or not I would go home. It was a long, long night.

Chapter 36

My alarm went off just as the sun was beginning to rise. It was time to leave. I had lived the past four months in a constant state of anxiety, but kissing Blaine goodbye and forcing myself to walk out that door was without a doubt one of the worst moments. The lights were still low in the hall while the nurses were going through shift change. The night nurse happened to be briefing the incoming day nurse right outside Blaine's door, and I updated them both on all the things I had thought of through the night. They smiled at me sympathetically and promised to take extra good care of him. There was nothing left to do but leave. My feet had turned to concrete blocks, but I forced myself to put one in front of the other, knowing each step was taking me further away from Blaine, not knowing with complete certainty if I would see him again.

One step led to another, and before I knew it, I was standing outside the hospital. I blinked rapidly as my burning eyes tried to adjust to the sunshine. I had not been outdoors in eight days. A light breeze touched my skin, and birds twittered to each other as I walked to the parking garage. I remembered racing into the hospital to escape the approaching hurricane the last time I had been outside, and now the weather was perfect . . . hot, but otherwise perfect.

I climbed into the Mustard Seed, our nickname for the borrowed yellow Kia Soul we were driving, and tried to mentally prepare myself for the massive amount I was about to be charged to get out of the garage. I hadn't prepared myself enough. I stared blankly at the screen showing "$120," trying to come up with a way to avoid paying but eventually gave up and put in my card. I made a mental note never to mention that to Blaine and then drove back to the Cottage.

Bob and Melany, Blaine's father and stepmother, were waiting for me. They hugged me tightly, and I let myself sink into them. I felt my eyes well up with tears and considered breaking down completely now that someone else was there to care for Blaine, but there was no time for that, so I held it together. We chatted for a few minutes, and then I quickly threw a few things into my bag and we headed for the airport. They dropped me off at the door and went back to the Cottage to wait for visiting hours. Only one of them would be allowed in to see Blaine and only for a few hours a day, but it was better than nothing.

I made it through security without any problems and went in search of Starbucks. I seemed to be walking through a thick haze, as if I were dreaming. Surely a good dose of caffeine would take care of me. I walked up to the counter and asked for my go-to drink.

"I'm sorry. We're all out of coffee."

Obviously, I really wasn't quite awake.

"I'm sorry. What?"

"We're all out of coffee."

And there it was. Starbucks was out of coffee at 9:30 in the morning. Maybe I really was dreaming. I knew I wasn't, but you really have to wonder how the rest of your day is going to go if Starbucks has no coffee. I remembered seeing another restaurant a little ways back, so I headed there. Thankfully, they were able to provide me with my caffeine fix, as well as some actual food, which I remembered I needed, and I went to sit down at my gate. I still felt as if I were moving through a weird fog, but the caffeine did make me feel a little more together. Soon it was time to board and an hour-and-a-half later, I was back in Springfield.

I walked out of the airport, and my friend Sheri pulled up next to the curb. I jumped in, and she hugged me and then handed me a container of

Chick-Fil-A mac and cheese. "Oh my gosh! You didn't!" I exclaimed as I ripped off the lid and savored the cheesy goodness. I had mentioned in a post several days earlier that the Chick-Fil-A in the hospital was closed and I was craving it.

"I did." She grinned. "Welcome home!"

She dropped me off at the house, and I ran inside to wrap my arms around my girls. I just held them for the longest time, savoring the feeling. It felt so good to be home, but it felt so awful to be there without Blaine. Fear tried to settle over me like a blanket, but I fought it off. I had no control over whether or not Blaine would make it home. All I could control was how I used my time with the girls, and I was determined not to waste a second.

We chatted for a while and then drove over to the neighboring town to watch Kamryn's friend Zach play in one of his last football games. I tried to soak in all the sensations of doing something normal. I knew Blaine would have loved it, and my heart ached when I let myself think about his missing it, so I shoved those thoughts down and focused on just enjoying the moment.

Soon my phone rang. It was Melany. My heart skipped a beat. That couldn't be good. "Hello?" I answered. It was a little hard to hear over the crowd.

"Blaine's fine." She knew I'd be worried she was calling when I had planned to be at the game. "Unfortunately, I'm lost." After hearing about the crazy charges to park at the hospital, they had decided she would just drop Bob off for the visiting hours and then go back and pick him up when they were over. Somehow, she had taken a wrong turn going back to the Cottage. Thankfully, I had learned my way around quite well by then and was able to help her get back to a familiar road. We said goodbye, and I put my focus back on the game.

A little while later, she called back. She sounded shaken. "I accidentally backed into Lydia's neighbor." She paused and took a breath. "And I was driving your friend's car."

I confirmed she was okay physically and then listened to her story. She had passed Lydia's driveway, so she pulled into the next one. She looked around and no one was coming, so she put the car in reverse and backed out onto the street. *Crash!* The neighbor across the street had been backing out at the same time, and somehow neither one of them had seen the other. Thankfully no one was hurt, but it certainly made Bob and Melany's time in Texas even more stressful.

The next morning, I knew I needed to call Debbie and tell her about the car. The insurance company would be calling, and I didn't want her to be surprised. I felt nauseated as I dialed her number. They had so graciously lent us that car for four weeks. We had already kept it for twelve, and I had no idea when we would be able to return it. Now we had wrecked it. The damage was small, but I still felt so bad! I forced myself to dial her number. She was clearly happy to hear from me. I chatted for a few minutes and then plunged in. "So . . . Debbie. I'm afraid I have some bad news."

"Oh? What's the matter?"

"My mother-in-law was driving Faith's car yesterday and accidentally backed into someone. There's not a lot of damage, but there is some. I'm so sorry!"

"Was anyone hurt?"

"No."

"Okay. It's fine. Don't worry about it. These things happen. We'll just get it fixed when you get back."

My whole body relaxed. Truthfully, I expected her to react this way, but it was reassuring to hear it. Instead of adding to my stress, Debbie reminded me that physical possessions don't really matter and freed me to keep my attention on what does.

The next few days flew by. Blaine was finally released from the hospital. Bob and Melany did a fantastic job taking care of him, and he felt a little stronger each day. I focused on covering the girls with as much love as I possibly could and soaked up what they were giving me in return. I also took time to see a couple of friends. One morning, I met Traci at our coffee shop, and I filled her in on everything Blaine had been through the last few weeks. Eventually, she interrupted me and said, "You know, when all of this is over, you're really going to have to focus on taking care of yourself."

I paused, staring at her for a moment. When this was over, I was expecting to have to focus on getting Blaine healthier. "What do you mean? I'm fine," I dismissed her concern with a wave of my hand.

Traci sighed. "This is harder on you than you are realizing now. At the very least, I can almost promise you're going to have adrenal fatigue when it's over." I knew she was speaking from experience. She had helped her husband fight his brain tumor for years and then had to bury him and somehow move on with her life, but my situation was different. It was stressful, sure, but we had the assurance of knowing Blaine *probably* wouldn't die. "Just promise me you'll pay attention to yourself and do what you need to do to take care of you." I assured her I would, but deep down, I was sure if I could just get him back home and get back to our normal life, everything would be fine.

Chapter 37

The next day, before the sun was even up, I found myself back on a plane headed for Houston. I was scheduled to land at 8:15, but by that time, Blaine would have already undergone lab work, a chest X-ray, and even an MRI. The day before, his lab work had shown his phosphorus was critically low once again, and he had been at the hospital late that night getting an IV infusion, and then had to turn around and be there early in the morning to start his tests. I knew he, as well as Bob and Melany, were going to be exhausted, and I was anxious to get back to help.

I grabbed an Uber from the airport back to the Cottage and ran in to see Blaine. He still looked rough, but he was vertical and smiling, a huge improvement since I had seen him last. We all visited for just a bit, but soon it was time for Bob and Melany to start the long trek home. I was so thankful they had come! I wished there were more time to sit and talk with them, but I knew they were facing a long drive, and I was happy they were able to get a reasonably early start.

Blaine and I relaxed for a few hours, but soon it was time for his appointment with Dr. Baldyga. I couldn't wait to see his MRI! You could visually see Lumpy was even smaller now than it had been for the last MRI, so I was excited to hear the official results. I was also anxious to hear how Blaine's platelets were doing. I knew they needed to be at least 100 for them to start the chemo the next day. Yesterday they were 18. They had made the jump in time to start the last cycle on schedule, and I was expecting them to do it again, but it would be good to know for sure. Or maybe I wanted them to give him a break and put it off a few more days. I couldn't quite decide what I was hoping for.

Dr. Baldyga walked into the room beaming. "Mr. and Mrs. Parker! I have amazing news for you again!" She pushed a few keys on her computer and brought up that day's image of Lumpy next to the last image and the one done the day before his first round of chemo. Even I could clearly see it was markedly smaller. The chemo was working! "This is the good news. The bad news is your platelets are having trouble rebounding."

"Where are they?" I asked.

"Nineteen."

That was a long way from 100.

"Take the weekend to rest. We'll run labs again on Monday morning, and if they're high enough, we'll start treatment then. If not, we'll try again on Wednesday."

We thanked her and went back to the Cottage. While I was disappointed to have the schedule delayed, I was thankful his body would have a few more days to heal before the next round of poison. He was moving so slowly and seemed very unsteady on his feet. I suppose that's to be expected if your blood counts are as messed up as his were, but it was still very unnerving to need to walk right next to my normally big, strong husband so I could catch him if he fell.

Blaine lay down on the bed as soon as we walked through the door of the Cottage. It had been a big day for him! I lay down next to him and fiddled around online while he dozed. Sometime later, I noticed he was staring at me. "The MRI today was awful. I don't want to do that again."

"Really?" By this point, he had undergone several MRIs, and he had always said they were no big deal. "What happened?"

"I don't know. I just felt very . . . scared. Now I can't stop thinking about it. I don't want to do it again."

I had known Blaine for twenty-seven years, and I honestly cannot remember his ever saying he was scared of anything. "I don't think you'll need another one until right before surgery. That's a long time from now. Try not to worry about it." He nodded and went back to sleep, but now I was worried. Why would an MRI bother him? All he had to do was lie there. It was very strange.

It would get stranger. Over the next few days, Blaine became afraid of everything. He needed me to be in the room with him at all times, and he would get extremely upset at just the slightest bit of bad news. We had taken to watching episodes of *Little House on the Prairie* every day while we ate our lunch, but we frequently had to turn it off because what was happening on the screen was too stressful for him. He told me it was like a horror movie was playing in his head. He constantly saw images of awful things, and he couldn't turn them off. He had trouble focusing enough to read, but I introduced him to sudoku games on the iPad in an effort to help his brain think about something other than the horror scenes. This did help while he was actually playing, but as soon as he stopped, the movie track would start in his head again.

While Blaine was in the hospital, Mike had finally succeeded in getting rid of the racoons. I told myself he took them to live at a happy little farm. Maybe not, but I made a point of not asking. We really did miss them, but there was lots of other wildlife around the Cottage to keep us entertained. Every day, we loved watching the butterflies and hummingbirds and little lizards. What we didn't love were the roaches. It turns out Texas has the biggest roaches I've ever seen, and I've seen some big roaches. They are wood roaches, not cockroaches, but I still hated those suckers! Each one seemed to be approximately the size of a puppy and had a look of pure evil.

One day I saw one scampering across the kitchen floor, and I ran over to stomp on it as fast as I could. Just as I raised my foot, set on sending the roach back to hell where it belonged, the puppy-sized devil's spawn flew straight at me! I take great pride in my country roots. I am no stranger to bugs. They don't bother me. I am calm, cool, and collected. I am a mature adult.

Or so I thought. The giant demon-bug flew in my direction, and I lost it completely. "Aaaaaaarrrrgggghhhhhhh!" I waved my arms and danced around in a circle.

Blaine's head shot up. "What's the matter?"

"The roaches fly!" I screamed as I continued to dance around, certain it had somehow infected me with its devil juice.

Blaine laughed. I paused, momentarily wondering if the trauma had been worth it to hear him laugh. Nope. It wasn't.

I rushed over to where it had landed and sent it to its final demise with one stomp of my foot. I then tried to determine just how scalding of a shower I needed, even though, truthfully, it hadn't even come close to touching me. Slowly my heart rate returned to normal, and I went on with my day, but my war with those roaches would continue.

Chapter 38

Around this time, the text came that I had been dreading. Our friend Bradley passed away. Tears ran down my cheeks as I read Elesha's text. I was sick to my stomach as I imagined how she must be feeling. The realization that I needed to tell Blaine also made me sick. He couldn't handle watching something sad happen to a fictional character on a TV show. I was really afraid he would break down completely with the news that someone he cared about, who had faced the same battle he was currently facing, had lost. It took me several days to build up the courage to give him the news. When I finally did, he surprised me. He obviously was very sad, but it didn't break him. Cancer is awful, and there's just no way around it.

Time kept marching on, and soon the weekend was over and it was time to see if Blaine's platelets had risen to the 100 mark. It was also our wedding anniversary! This obviously was not the way I would have ever hoped to spend our anniversary, but I was determined to make the best of it. We started the day with an early trip to the lab, hoping to get the news that Blaine's counts were at acceptable levels and he could start the fifth cycle of chemo. The waiting room was always very crowded, but on this day, it seemed like half of Houston was there at the same time. Finally, it was his turn to go back. They took what they needed, and we headed back to the Cottage to wait for the results, fully expecting to drive back in a couple of hours to start his infusion.

That was not going to happen. Soon after arriving home, the email came notifying me that his results had been posted. I opened the link as fast as I could and scanned through all the numbers until I came to his platelets.

Sixty.

"Shoot."

Blaine was working across the table from me. I hadn't meant to say that out loud. "What's the matter?"

There was no use sugar coating it. "Your platelets are only at 60." I quickly scanned through the rest of his results. "Everything else looks decent, though."

A little while later, Dr. Baldyga's nurse called to tell us what we already knew. Sixty was much better than 19, but still a long way from 100. She said they'd check again in two days, and hopefully he could get started then.

I spent the rest of our anniversary working. Blaine alternated between working and napping. He still felt pretty lousy. Even if he felt well, it wouldn't have been safe for him to go anywhere with his depressed immune system and the COVID germs everywhere. That evening, I celebrated by ordering a nice dinner to be delivered. Blaine drank a delicious container of Ensure. I rambled on about how much better the next anniversary would be and silently prayed over and over that I was right.

The next two weeks crept by. Every other day we would go to the hospital so they could check on Blaine's platelets. Each time I would anxiously wait for the results to be posted, certain they would reach the magic number, and then I would be disappointed. They went up a couple of points every day, but nowhere close to the threshold where they needed to be. I begged God to fix them. I wanted so desperately to move forward so we could go home.

Obviously, I wanted this time to be over so we could go back to our girls and to our real life, but there was another problem that loomed like a dark shadow creeping closer and closer in my mind—our deductible. We had met our $16,000 family out-of-pocket deductible during our first week in Texas, and for the rest of the year, all of his treatment was free, but if anything carried over into January, we would start all over. In addition to two more cycles of chemotherapy, he was still facing weeks of radiation and then the surgery with the long hospital stay. Everything needed to be timed out perfectly in order to have the possibility of its being wrapped up by the end of the year. I was already fighting so hard to keep my brain from panicking about our bills. The thought that we could possibly start it all completely over for the next year made me feel like I was sliding down a deep, dark hole I might never climb out of.

So, I prayed and prayed and prayed for what I wanted. I wanted Blaine to be cured. I wanted his treatment to move forward. I wanted everything to be done by December 31. Then slowly, I realized what I should want was what God wanted. I knew ultimately God's plan was best; He knew things I didn't, and I really just needed to trust Him . . . but that was so hard! I've faced big problems in the past, and God has always, always come through for me, in better ways than I had even dreamed. I knew all of that in my heart, but it was so hard to completely trust Him, knowing that in the short term, His plan might look very different from mine.

During this week, we passed the three-month anniversary of our being in Houston. While I had been able to make a few trips home, it had been ninety days since Blaine had seen his children, slept in his own bed, or sat at his desk and joked with his coworkers. Three whole months. My mind kept going back to the night we told the girls he had cancer. We had assured them it was no big deal and would quickly be taken care of. We were completely honest with them. We just had no idea what was coming. I now understood that our ignorance had really been God's protection. If He had allowed us to know what our future held, I don't know how we could have handled it. I thought back to being told we needed to stay in Houston for a week for the initial tests and being completely baffled as to how we would make that work. I worried about the girls' staying home by themselves for a whole week. I worried about how we would cover all the expenses involved with being away that long. I worried about Blaine's job. I worried about mine. They all seemed like such big problems at the time.

Part of me was overwhelmed with gratitude at how God had taken care of us through all of this, all of the ways He had met our needs. I truthfully was so thankful, but part of me was really scared. If He had sheltered us from the knowledge of what was to come, how did I know He wasn't still doing that? How did I know there wasn't some awful thing headed our way that He was protecting us from knowing about now?

Chapter 39

Eventually, enough time passed that Dr. Baldyga was confident Blaine's platelets would be at the magic threshold to finally begin the fifth round of chemo. We had been instructed to have his blood drawn early the next morning and then go immediately to the infusion center to get started. I knew it would be a long day, and I knew I needed to be well rested to face it.

Instead of sleeping though, I lay awake in a total panic for hours. We had learned that instead of bringing the doxorubicin home and having it infuse over several days, it was common to administer it super-fast over a few minutes, instead. Some doctors believed that lowered the chance of the patient suffering sores afterward. There was some data that suggested it carried a slightly higher risk of heart damage, but Dr. Baldyga thought that risk was minimal enough to make it worth trying. We had agreed while we were sitting in her nice, safe exam room, but now that it was almost time to actually do it, I was so terrified I thought *I* might suffer heart damage.

I knew I needed to pray, but I was afraid. Our biggest prayer during this entire ordeal had been that Dr. Baldyga would know exactly how Blaine's specific cancer needed to be treated, but she would not even consider deviating from the standard treatment protocol of six rounds of chemo. During the last chemo cycle, I had fasted and prayed that Blaine wouldn't have any side effects, and he ended up with the worst ones to date. While he had been on the holding floor, the nurse had prayed such a seemingly Spirit-filled prayer for him that I was sure he must have been cured right then, but instead his fever spiked a few hours later, and he ended up in the hospital for twelve days, sicker than anyone I had ever seen. Now I had prayed for good rest, and instead I was wide awake, freaking out over everything. It seemed that God was doing the exact opposite of what I was asking. I knew I should be praying about the infusion the next day, but I was too afraid to do it.

Soon, my alarm went off, and it was time to get moving. We went to the lab and then upstairs to wait for the official word that he was safe to start. We were sitting in the waiting room when my phone rang. I answered and was surprised to hear Dr. Baldyga's voice. Before, one of her nurses had always delivered her messages to me.

"So . . . ," she began. "Blaine's platelets are only at 87."

My heart sank. Eighty-seven! We should be nearing the time of starting the sixth cycle, and we hadn't even started the fifth.

She went on, "I don't think we should wait any longer. It's time to stop the chemo and move on with his radiation and surgery."

My mind was reeling with the fact that the platelets were still so low, but I knew I needed to focus on what she was saying. Obviously, I had missed something.

"I'm sorry. What did you say?"

"It is time to stop the chemo. His body is not responding well. We need to move forward with the radiation and then the surgery."

"You want to stop the chemo?" I didn't think Blaine was listening to this conversation, but his head whipped toward me, his eyes huge.

"Yes."

"You're saying he's done?" Blaine's eyes got even bigger.

"After his surgery, we will determine whether or not he needs the last two cycles, but for now he is done. We will notify the radiation oncologist that he is ready to begin. You need to go to the vascular department and have them remove the CVC. We will let them know you're coming."

I was dumbfounded. I stumbled over my words as I thanked her and hung up the phone. I told Blaine what she had said, and we both just sat there, too shocked by the abrupt change in plans to move. "What if she's wrong?" Blaine whispered.

I didn't know how to answer him. What if she *was* wrong? "She's not," I said resolutely so Blaine would know I was totally confident she had made the right decision, even though I was terrified she hadn't. "Let's go. It will be so nice to get the CVC line out. You can take a real shower!"

I grabbed our bag and stood up. Blaine didn't move. "What if they just have to put it right back in? Maybe I should just keep it."

"They won't," I assured him, even though I had almost zero confidence that was true. "It's going to be awesome." I planted a huge smile on my face. "The worst is over!" I pulled him up, and we started for the vascular department.

A few minutes later, we were on the skywalk tram to the main building where the vascular department is located when the realization of what had just happened hit me like a ton of bricks. I had been so upset that God seemed to be answering my prayers in the exact opposite way of what I wanted, when the truth was He had been working all along to answer my biggest prayer.

While I had been praying so hard Blaine wouldn't have any side effects from the chemo, God was busy using those side effects to actually meet our greatest need. I thought God was ignoring my pleas, but He was actually doing exactly what was best for Blaine. On her own, there was no way Dr. Baldyga was going to deviate from the basic treatment plan. It took Blaine's body reacting so badly to the chemotherapy for her to stop it. We had been praying so hard that she would know exactly how much chemo was needed to kill all of the cancer cells. I could suddenly clearly see that he needed four cycles and how God had made it plain to her that it was time to stop. If he hadn't reacted badly, she would have given him two more rounds, and who knows what damage they would have caused?

We checked in at the vascular department. They had been expecting us and got us back in a room quickly. Both of us kept fidgeting with our clothes and giving each other worried glances. Putting the CVC line in had been a big deal. We assumed taking it out would be as well and were shocked when they let me go back in the room with him. The nurse was getting things ready as Blaine lay down on the exam table. "How hard is it to get this thing out?" I asked.

"Oh! Not hard at all!" She turned around, wiped his skin down with an alcohol pad, fiddled with the tube for a moment, and then just pulled the whole thing out. I doubt the entire process took five seconds. We couldn't believe it! She held it up. "All done!" she announced.

"That's it?" Blaine asked. His relief was palpable.

"That's it! Have a great day!"

We thanked her and started the long walk back to the car. The drive to the Cottage was quiet. We were both numb. I couldn't believe how quickly everything had changed! We had left that morning completely expecting to spend the whole day in the hospital getting his chemo infusion, knowing that it was necessary but likely to make him deathly ill. Instead, we were home before lunch, his body free of implanted medical devices and our future looking bright. The worst was truly over!

The second I walked through the door of the Cottage, I felt as if every ounce of energy I ever had were sucked right out of me! I had been so pumped up just a few minutes earlier! I managed to text the girls and post a message to his Facebook group updating them with the big news and then told Blaine I needed to take a nap. I lay down on the bed and instantly fell asleep. Three hours later, I finally woke up, refreshed and filled with an overwhelming sense of joy. I felt a little guilty, and dumb, for doubting God was taking care of Blaine, but it was such an amazing feeling to know so clearly that He had been all along!

Chapter 40

Two days later, we found ourselves in the radiation section of the hospital. Blaine had been there during his initial visit, but it was my first time. I was so anxious to hear their plan! During Blaine's initial consultation, Dr. Gancio, the radiation oncologist, had said he would need five weeks of radiation treatments. Lumpy was now so much smaller, and the MRI showed "dramatically diminished internal enhancement," so I was sure he wouldn't need that many. Somehow, I just knew he only needed three weeks. I thought he would start receiving the treatments the next day and in three weeks, we would be on our way home!

Dr. Gancio and her student walked into the room, said hello to Blaine, and introduced themselves to me. Their obvious concern for Blaine's well-being was clear, and I immediately felt as if they were both my friends.

Soon, I liked them a little less. "We will take measurements today for the brace that will hold your arm in place for the radiation. That will only take a week to be built, and then we can get started."

It was going to take a week just to get started! That was very disappointing, but at least we would be going home three weeks after that.

I decided maybe I should just get that fact clarified for sure. "And how many treatments will he need?"

"Only twenty-five! In just six weeks he'll be all done!"

My heart fell. I'm certain my face did also. Six weeks! We talked about the fact that Lumpy was so much smaller, and theoretically "deader," but it didn't change the plan. The team had met and decided twenty-five radiation treatments had the best chance of ensuring all cancer cells around Lumpy were obliterated before surgery. The more we talked, the more I decided I liked them again, even though I was disappointed with their plan.

They took us down to the radiation room and showed us all around, explaining the process to both of us. Then Dr. Gancio and I left the room so the technicians could begin the radiation simulation, in which they calibrated the perfect positioning for Blaine's arm in order for the laser to hit exactly the right spot. They put tiny tattoos on his skin so they would know exactly where to line up the laser. They also made a mold for the device that would hold his arm in place. This is what would take a week to build.

During the week we were waiting for the immobilization device to be built for the radiation, it was finally time for Blaine's appointment with the dermatologist. Blaine was still feeling pretty awful, and the walk from the parking garage to the dermatology department was exhausting. When his name was finally called, he shuffled back to the room and sat down heavily on the table. The student asked him to take off his shirt so she could examine him. He did and then just sat there looking old and miserable.

Usually, his appearance didn't shock me much by this point, but every now and then I would see him with fresh eyes, and I would be totally taken aback. He actually reminded me of pictures I have seen of prisoners in concentration camps. He was completely bald; his skin just hung on his frame, and his eyes usually had a vacant look, like he really just did not care what happened to him next.

The student looked at the spots we had been concerned about and actually found a few new ones we hadn't mentioned and then sent a message to the physician that she was ready for him. I watched as he and the student examined Blaine's skin closely. To my horror, I noticed a small drop of mucus began to form at the end of Blaine's nostril. The awful sores from the mucositis had finally cleared up, but the excessive mucus was still an issue.

They continued to look over Blaine's body while the drop got bigger . . . and bigger. I was not sure if Blaine even knew it was there. His normal self would have been completely mortified. The drop got bigger . . . and bigger. I didn't know what to do. I was afraid I would upset Blaine if I said something, but I didn't want him to be embarrassed if it fell. It got bigger . . . and bigger. I honestly couldn't believe it was still hanging on!

Finally, the doctor reached over and grabbed a tissue and very nonchalantly handed it to Blaine, like mucus fell out of his patients' noses every day, which it probably did. Blaine seemed a little surprised but just wiped it off, and they went on with their exam.

"I'm sure the spots on your shoulder and your face are fine, but I am pretty concerned about this," he said as he pointed to a spot on Blaine's arm, "and this," as he pointed to a spot on his back. "We need to get those biopsied today."

I just stared at him for a moment, trying to force my mind to comprehend what he had said. Just as Blaine was finishing the worst part of the cancer treatment and things were finally looking up, now he potentially had a completely different type of cancer? After my last trip home, I had a conversation with the Uber driver about his grandmother, who had been treated at MDA for two types of cancer at the same time, one of them being skin cancer. I remember thinking how awful it would be to have to fight two simultaneously, and now that was potentially going to be our reality. The fact that his grandmother had died was not helping my anxiety.

The doctor left the student to take the biopsies from both spots. The process looked painful, but Blaine just sat there, looking defeated. As awful as it was for me to wrap my head around the fact that we may be starting a brand-new battle, I couldn't even imagine how hard it was for Blaine! She put Band-Aids on both spots and instructed us to keep the areas moist with an antibiotic cream. "I'll call you as soon as I have the results, but they will probably take about a week." I was hoping she would look optimistic and cheerful as she talked. She didn't.

We went back to the Cottage and just went on like things were normal. Blaine worked a little and napped a lot. We didn't talk about it with each other, and I didn't breathe a word of it to anyone else. Part of me was afraid mentioning it would somehow make it real, but part of me worried people would start to get tired of hearing about all our problems. Seriously, how much trouble could one family have? I was concerned people would think we were making things up.

The week crept by so slowly! Once again, we were just waiting—waiting for the radiation to start and waiting to hear if Blaine had skin cancer. Thankfully, he felt a little stronger every day. We started walking laps back and forth between the Cottage and the big house. It was no longer so hot I feared our skin would melt off, and it was good for Blaine to get some fresh air and a little exercise. Every day he would push himself to walk a few more laps. One day he announced he would like to walk on the road. He made it all the way to the end of the block, and I couldn't stop beaming at him! He was very slow, a little unsteady, and had to wipe the mucus that continued to drip from his nose every few minutes, but he made it!

It felt so strange to be living in this weird little vacuum in which our life was the same every day while everyone else's was moving on normally. The night of Kamryn's homecoming dance arrived. She had a great time, and Kaci and Zach's mom kept me updated with pictures so I wouldn't feel completely left out. I hated so much that I was missing it, but the updates did help, and the knowledge that the end of our time in Texas was in sight, assuming Blaine didn't have skin cancer, helped too. Hopefully this would be the last major life event I would have to miss!

Exactly a week after the dermatology appointment, I was sitting at the kitchen table trying to get some work done when my phone vibrated. I casually glanced down to see who it was. The screen read, "MDA Dermatology." My breath caught, and I held it. I knew they must be calling with the results of Blaine's skin biopsies, but I was afraid to hear what they had to say. My hands were shaking as I forced myself to answer. I was sweating, and it seemed as if my heart had stopped beating while I waited. Thankfully, she was quick. "I have great news for you, Mrs. Parker!" she said. I let out my breath, and my heart started beating again. "Both of the biopsies of Blaine's skin came back as melanocytic nevi." I tried desperately to guess what these words meant but had no idea. Thankfully, she went on. "They're both completely benign lesions and nothing at all to worry about."

"Oh! Thank you for calling! Is there anything else he needs to do?"

"Just keep putting the antibiotic cream on them until they heal, but that's all. There's no reason to come back in."

I thanked her again, then hung up and gave Blaine the good news. Then I went to take a nap. Exactly like when we learned the chemo treatments were over, I was again immediately completely exhausted. I fell into the bed, closed my eyes, and was asleep before I knew it. Two hours later I awoke feeling completely refreshed and ready to tackle the next few weeks!

Chapter 41

The next day was Blaine's first official radiation appointment. Dr. Gancio, her student, and the technicians had prepared us well, but we were still pretty nervous. The radiation department of the hospital felt like a whole different world. There was even a separate entrance for patients receiving radiation treatments. I pulled into the horseshoe driveway and was relieved to see there were cars in front of me. We had been told there was valet parking for radiation patients, but I was not sure how the process worked. We drove up under the covered area and watched as the driver and patient in front of us got out of their car, said a few words to the employee, took a ticket, and walked into the hospital.

When it was our turn, I pulled up to the spot and stepped out of the car. A young man with a heavy accent and a clipboard asked for the patient's name.

"Blaine Parker."

He scanned down his list, found Blaine's name, and put a mark next to it. As he tore off my ticket, he said, "I see it's your first time here. Welcome to the radiation department!" I couldn't exactly place his accent, but it was delightful and somehow made me feel almost jolly. "We'll take care of your car. Go inside and down the stairs. Hand the ladies at the desk this ticket, and they'll validate that your husband is here to receive radiation. When he's finished, bring us back this ticket, and we'll bring back your car. Easy peasy!" he said with a huge grin.[11]

I thanked him and took my ticket, and we walked through the doors into a tropical oasis. Sunlight streamed through the floor-to-ceiling windows nourishing the many plants as well as the patients waiting inside. We went down the stairs and immediately came to a desk with more smiling faces. The ladies behind the desk stamped our parking ticket and gave Blaine an ID card that he was to bring with him every time he came for treatment. Then they told Blaine which room he was assigned to that day and pointed us in the direction we should go.

Each step took us further and further down into the catacombs of the hospital. No wonder they had put so much effort into making the entry pleasant! The hallway twisted and turned as we seemed to move further and further underground. The flickering fluorescent lights cast eerie shadows, and I held my breath as we went around every corner. Somehow, we had stumbled into a 1970s horror movie.

We finally arrived at his assigned waiting room. We were still underground, so obviously there were no windows, but they had done the best they could to make it pleasant. Comfortable chairs invited us to sit, and nature photographs decorated the walls. Blaine scanned his new ID card into the computer, which let the technicians know he was ready. Soon they came to get him, and I settled into a chair to wait.

All of his radiation appointments were conveniently scheduled in the early morning so he could work the rest of the day. I was the only one in the waiting room at first, but soon other patients, and in some cases their caregivers, started to trickle in. Over the next five weeks, these people would become our world. There was the football coach with rectal cancer, the young mom juggling supporting her sick mother with raising her own children, the realtor with a brain tumor who was so scared, and the blind man who was fighting his third type of cancer, supported by his wife and guide dog. Sometimes our schedules weren't exactly the same, but most days we could count on seeing "our" people, and they provided the support and familiarity that we desperately needed.

Blaine told me that every day as they walked him back to the radiation room, they officially confirmed his identity, even though they knew exactly who he was since they saw him every day. When they arrived to the room, there were two or three technicians already there, and they would always have his favorite type of music playing. They would all chat for a few minutes about all of their lives, and then they would get started.

Blaine would remove his shirt and take everything out of his pockets and then lie down on the hard table. They would ask if he had any questions or concerns and check the skin around Lumpy to see how it was holding up to the radiation. On the first day, one of the techs marked Blaine's arm with a green marker to make it easier to aim the laser at exactly the correct spots. They covered the marks with clear tape to keep the ink from rubbing off, but every day they would need to mark these again and reapply the tape. Then they would put his arm into the form that had been built to hold it in place. While one tech was doing this, another would position the laser just right.

When it was set, they would dim the lights and leave the room. Blaine would hear clicks and a hum from the machine and knew to lie very still. Approximately five minutes later, the machine would turn off, the lights would come on, and the technicians would come back into the room. One would retract the laser; one would help him sit up and get off the table; one would return the arm form to its storage location, and one would start sanitizing the table. Blaine would put his shirt back on; they would all say goodbye, and then one of the techs would escort him back to the waiting area and call the next patient. They would chat about everything from Houston's pothole problem to the fall of the Berlin Wall, and Blaine quickly grew to love them.

The first appointment or two took a little longer, but once they had everything set just right, most days we would be in and out, from dropping our car off with the valet guys to picking it back up again, within twenty minutes or less. Every single staff person we encountered there was friendly and smiling, and the entire department seemed to run like clockwork. Within minutes of Blaine swiping his card, a technician would come to get him, sometimes even a few minutes before his scheduled appointment time. They would make him feel comfortable, administer the radiation perfectly, and then send him on his way. I've never experienced any other medical office nearly as efficient as they were, and I was impressed every single day.

The day we learned we needed to be in Houston six more weeks for the radiation, I got online and booked a flight for Kaci and Kamryn to fly down. Kaia was not able to miss class or practice, but the other two were able to adjust their schedules fairly easily. I was so excited! It had been several weeks since I was home, but poor Blaine hadn't seen them for months! I had guessed at the earliest possible date Blaine would be strong enough to be around other people, and it worked out perfectly. As expected, he had been feeling a little bit stronger every day, and although his white count still wasn't normal, it was high enough the doctors all felt he would be fine for the girls to come—as long as they didn't have COVID, of course.

The day of their flight finally arrived. Our friend Sharon had graciously offered to drive them to the airport and had even bought at-home COVID tests for them to take first. I was so nervous one of their tests would be positive but soon received the text I had been waiting for: "We're negative and on our way!" All of a sudden, everything was fine. Blaine was feeling better, and in just a few hours, most of our family would be together!

The girls had never flown by themselves, and I was just a little bit nervous for them, but they made it through security without any problems, and soon they were settled at their gate, just waiting to board the plane. I had made cookies for them, and the whole Cottage smelled delicious, as if even it were looking forward to their arrival. Blaine and I were trying to focus on our work but kept checking the time to see how much longer it would be before we could leave for the airport to get them.

At some point, my phone rang, and I looked down to discover Kaci was calling. I grabbed it as fast as I could. "Hi, Sweetie!"

"I think our flight's been canceled."

I could feel my heart sinking. "Why do you think that?"

"Because they just announced it over the intercom, and now everyone is leaving here and going to the desk."

That seemed like a pretty good reason.

I told her to follow them and find out what was going on. She soon called back and confirmed that the flight had indeed been canceled—no reason given, they just weren't going to fly that day. They refunded our money but couldn't fix our disappointment. The airline was small and only flew on certain days, so it was going to be a full week before their trip could be rescheduled. The gloom settled back over us again, but there was nothing to do but move forward. They called Sharon, who graciously came back to take them home, and Blaine and I finished our work for the day.

I ate all their cookies.

Chapter 42

The next day, Blaine was standing at the sink washing off a dish. He turned around to tell me something and suddenly gasped and grabbed his side. "What's wrong?" I asked, trying not to sound as panicked as I felt.

"I don't know. I just felt this awful electrical shock. It's gone now. It was just for a second, but it hurt like crazy."

We tried not to think too much about it, but several times a day, at completely random moments, he would feel as if someone were shocking him with a Taser. The pain was in his side, not his arm, where the radiation was being directed, but near it. It only lasted for a second or two. Blaine has a very high pain tolerance, but he gasped and grabbed his side every time it came.

The shooting pains continued off and on through the weekend. I was thankful we had an appointment every Monday morning with Dr. Gancio. As expected, she didn't mess around and immediately ordered an ultrasound of the area. I was trying hard not to worry about what might be wrong, but of course my mind kept suggesting horrible possibilities.

The ultrasound came back completely normal—nothing at all unusual. I was so relieved! Unfortunately, that meant we still had no answer as to what was causing Blaine's pain. Dr. Gancio and her student got to work and figured out the area was indeed at the very edge of the radiation circle. The pain had to be coming from the radiation, even though they had never had a patient have that side effect before. It was odd it hurt there and not where the bulk of the radiation was hitting. He obviously needed the treatment, though, so there was no choice but to keep going.

Aside from the sporadic debilitating pain, overall Blaine was slowly becoming more and more himself. One night that week we were watching TV when he suddenly jumped up, ran across the room, and stomped his foot down hard on the floor. I just stared at him. He looked back at me and nonchalantly said, "Roach." He had killed one of the horrible devil's spawn for me! I ran over and hugged him. My hero was returning!

Finally, the day of the girls' new flight arrived. This time we all kept our excitement in check. Surely the flight wouldn't be canceled again, but we didn't want to get our hopes up. Sharon bought new COVID tests; they passed, and she drove them to the airport again. Blaine and I seemed to be holding our breath, but soon they sent a picture of their smiling, masked faces actually on the airplane!

We stayed at the Cottage as long as we could stand it but eventually left for the airport way too early. Time creeped by as we waited for their plane to land and then for them to make their way to us. Finally, we saw their faces pop around the corner, and a second later Blaine had wrapped them both up in the tightest bear hug he'd ever given.

He held them for a very long time, but eventually we headed for the car. I couldn't stop staring at them. I was sad Kaia could not be there but beyond thrilled most of us were together! I was looking forward to showing Kamryn and Kaci some sites around Houston, but mostly I was just excited that at least for a bit, life would feel a little more normal. The business of having our family living separately was so hard for me, but for a few days at least most of us would finally be together.

We had such a fun week! Every morning one of the girls would go with Blaine to his radiation appointment. The first time each of them went, the technicians gave them a tour and explained exactly what they were doing to their dad, and then they would go wait in the waiting area until he was done. The rest of the day, we would kill time around the Cottage while

Blaine worked, and then we explored the highlights of the city. I had made a big deal of how much I hated Houston, but truthfully, there are lots of lovely areas and fun things to do.

One day we went to the Health Museum, which had been recommended to us by one of the radiation nurses. We ambled slowly through the museum, trying out all the interactive displays. Kaci and I stopped to watch a short video while Blaine and Kamryn went ahead to explore the brain teaser area. The movie finished, and Kaci and I went to catch up with them. We walked around the corner and noticed everyone was crowded around Blaine. The lights may have been bouncing off his bald head, and his clothes may have been four sizes too big for his new body, but everyone in the room was listening intently to his instructions for solving the puzzles. Kamryn stood off to the side, beaming with pride. Four weeks ago, Blaine had not been able to comprehend more than one sentence at a time, but now he was once again the smartest person in the room! I made no attempt at all to stop the tears from running down my cheeks while I watched him. The change was almost unbelievable, and I was so grateful, I thought my heart would burst.

The week flew by, and I had to accept the fact the girls would leave us the next day. I made one final dinner for them and sadly sat down to watch Kaci check in for their fight. She clicked a few things on her phone and then paused. "Mom, you're not going to believe this. They canceled our flight!" She was right; I didn't believe it! They were able to get seats on a flight just a few days later, and I was thrilled we got to keep them a little longer.

We decided to make the most of the surprise extra time and venture out of Houston a bit—to the beach! Being from landlocked Missouri, going to the beach is a huge deal and the hour-long drive to Galveston was an easy choice. The girls and I were so excited. Somehow, Blaine does not like the beach, but he went along with us and was a good sport. We found him a rocking chair in the shade, and then the three of us went down to splash in the water.

I tried to soak in every moment. I wanted to always remember the girls' laughing faces, the way the sand felt on my toes, and the miracle of Blaine looking down at us in his body that had been through hell but was climbing back out. I stared at the vastness of the ocean and felt the truth that the same God who made it was watching over us, that He had given us this day at the beach, this joy in the middle of the awfulness.

As I sat in the sand and watched the girls run through the surf, I was reminded that life is always like this—ups and downs, awfulness and joy. Some days our hearts break, but then some days our hearts burst with bliss. On the days we're stuck in the yuck, we just have to trust that the joy-filled days are coming. They are. We just have to hang on until they get there. I closed my eyes and lifted my face to the sun, feeling the ocean spray and listening to my girls squeal as the freezing water rushed over their ankles. I locked the moment in my mind. I knew harder days were likely coming and I would need this reminder.

The next day, we took the girls to the airport. As they walked away from us, I kept my eyes glued on them until they were completely swallowed by the crowd. It felt much more significant than just watching them get on a plane. I missed them so much, and deep down, I was afraid things would never be exactly the same again.

Chapter 43

Over the next few weeks, Blaine and I fell into a comfortable routine. We got up in the morning and went for his treatment and then came home and worked the rest of the day. Before we started working, I rubbed emu oil all over Blaine's skin that was being hit with the radiation. We started this on the very first day—way before his skin showed any signs of being irritated. Every night before he went to sleep, I rubbed Aquaphor lotion on it. Lydia had recommended the emu oil, and the radiation staff had recommended the Aquaphor. The combination worked wonders! Dr. Gancio had warned us the type of radiation Blaine was receiving, while expected to do less damage internally, would likely burn his skin significantly. After five weeks of treatment, his skin was red and a little itchy, but he never had any blisters at all, and he said it didn't even hurt.

As soon as we knew what day Blaine was going to start radiation, I messaged his surgeon and asked if we could schedule the surgery. I knew there was now a good chance we could have everything wrapped up before the end of the year, and I didn't want to take a chance on messing that up because we hadn't gotten it on the calendar. The next day, they messaged back and told me his surgery was scheduled for December 16. They reminded me he would need to be in Houston the week before and for two weeks after. That put us heading home for good on December 30. My heart leaped into my throat. We had an end date! For so long my sister had been telling me every day was one day closer. Now I could finally count down the days! This also meant he would be done with the most expensive procedures before our deductible started over. I felt like such a weight had been lifted. We were going to make it!

Soon though, I realized the significance of the time between December 16 and 30: Christmas. We were going to be stuck in Texas for Christmas. It seemed crazy that we had to be away from home last year due to Kaia's COVID restrictions, and now we were going to have to be away from home again. I was obsessed with not spending any unnecessary money but having my family together for Christmas felt necessary, and I got online to check on flights for the girls.

To my shock, even though we were more than two months away from Christmas, there was only one seat left on the reasonably priced airline out of Des Moines on the date Kaia would be available to travel. That scared me, so I hurried and checked flights out of Springfield for Kaci and Kamryn. There were only two seats left! I couldn't believe my "luck"! I quickly booked all three and called the girls to tell them the plan. It wasn't as nice as being at home for Christmas, but at least we would all be together.

Now I had a new project: figuring out how to make Christmas away from home feel special without spending any money. I enjoyed researching different Christmas activities in Houston and reading posts about favorite traditions, but I just couldn't come up with any great ideas. After all the trauma of the last year, I wanted something that would be really amazing for the girls. I was discussing it one day casually with Lydia when she said, "Well, you're welcome to use our beach condo."

I just stared at her while my mind slowly absorbed what she had said. They owned a beach condo? We could actually spend Christmas on the beach? That was certainly better than any of my ideas. The girls would love it! Who was I kidding? *I* would love it! Blaine would not love it, but he would love that the rest of us were happy.

I finally remembered I needed to reply to her. "You own a beach condo? Are you sure you won't be using it?"

"Yes, we've owned it for years and it will just be sitting empty during Christmas. You're more than welcome to use it."

I hugged her. "Thank you! That will be *perfect*! I can't wait to tell the girls. They're going to be so excited!" I hugged her again and ran inside the Cottage to tell Blaine and to call the girls. As expected, everyone was thrilled! Lumpy would be gone; Blaine would be recovering, and our family would be together again. Throw in some ocean waves and flip-flops in December, and it was going to be the absolute perfect way to wrap up this mess of a year. Everything was going to be okay!

Now that Christmas was settled, I was back to just focusing on getting Blaine through each day. Every Monday, after his radiation treatment, he had an appointment with Dr. Gancio just so she could check his skin and make sure everything was progressing well. Before she came in, her nurse checked Blaine's weight and his vital signs. He stepped on the scale, and the nurse checked the number. "You're up a pound!" she announced. Normally, a pound is not that big of a deal, and *gaining* a pound is not usually something people cheer about, but when your husband loses forty-plus pounds in a matter of a few weeks, starting to move in the other direction is something to celebrate!

We moved into the exam room. I was busy texting the girls about the gained pound while the nurse was checking Blaine's vital signs. "All good," she said. My head jerked up as I realized I hadn't been paying attention. Ever since his first scary trip to the ER, I had obsessed over his vital signs. Somehow, we had magically crossed into a period when I knew he was okay and I didn't have to worry about every little thing. I stared at him in wonder. He was definitely getting better. He now had obvious facial hair, still patchy but clearly coming in strong, and the hair on his head was just beginning to poke up too. The human body is incredible, and watching Blaine's rebuild itself was nothing short of amazing.

Time kept marching on. Our routine every day was pretty much the same as the day before, but each day was bringing us closer and closer to the end. It was now November. The weather at home had turned cold and dreary, but it was spectacular in Houston! Enduring the days of sweltering temperatures was finally paying off. It seemed every day was the perfect temperature; the sun shone, and flowers bloomed everywhere.

The five weeks of radiation actually seemed to pass pretty quickly, and all of a sudden, it was Blaine's last day. I had cheered for other people as they rang the bell signifying they had completed their treatment, and I could hardly believe it was finally Blaine's turn! I waited anxiously while he finished up in the treatment room. Soon a tech came to get me. Phone in hand, ready to record every second, I rounded the corner to see Blaine standing by the brass bell that hangs on the wall, a beacon of hope for every cancer patient and the people who love them. A giant smile took over my entire face, and I fought to keep from bouncing up and down as I waited. It seemed surreal that the day had finally come! We had made it!

His entire radiation team came out to help him celebrate. I would have rung the bell as fast as I could, like a crazy person, but Blaine did it slow and steady, like a ship coming through the fog, which is really more symbolic of the whole experience. The techs all clapped for him. Our new friends in the waiting room clapped for him. It was a moment I will never forget.

Blaine said goodbye to all the techs. It was such an odd sensation—joy and sadness together simultaneously. He had seen these people every day for the last five weeks. They had helped him through the most difficult time in his life, and they had played a critical role in saving him. They had become his friends, and as happy as he was to be going home, I knew he would miss them.

We walked past the waiting area, and again, complete strangers whom we had bonded with through this shared nightmare cheered for us and told us goodbye. We all wished each other the best and promised to pray for each other. We kept walking through the hallway maze and eventually came to the check-in desk. The ladies there congratulated us and wished us well. It was so strange to know we would not make this trek again. Soon we were in the parking area. Our precious valets brought back the Mustard Seed and cheered for us as we got in. We thanked them for everything, and I drove away from the radiation section of the hospital for the very last time.

Chapter 44

One of the many problems with getting unexpectedly stuck in another state for six months is sometimes things expire—like your driver's license. We knew Blaine's renewal date was coming up but had expected to be home in plenty of time. I had tried to renew it over the phone but was denied. It really didn't matter. Blaine was too sick to drive most of the time, but now we were facing an eleven-hour trip. Six months ago, I would have been really concerned about driving all that way myself, but now it barely fazed me. I had discovered I was much more capable than I knew.

We packed up the car that evening and hit the road at 5:00 the next morning, hoping to get out of town before the traffic got bad. No such luck! I couldn't believe how many cars were on the road even before the sun came up, but we made it just fine, and driving the entire eleven hours was not nearly as bad as I had been expecting.

We finally pulled into the garage, and Kaci and Kamryn ran out to welcome us home. I rushed to unbuckle my seatbelt and jump out of the car almost before I put it in park. We took turns hugging each girl over and over and then went inside. I was a little worried about how the dogs would handle Blaine. They hadn't seen him in almost six months, and he looked vastly different than when he had left. I shouldn't have worried. The second they saw him, they went crazy, jumping and twisting, trying to get as close to him as they could. He knew for sure he had been missed!

Kaci had made us dinner, and as we sat down to eat, I tried to notice everything: the last of the day's sunlight streaming through my glass door, the look in Blaine's eyes as he realized the worst of his fight was over and he was finally home, the huge grin on both of the girls' faces with the knowledge they weren't alone anymore. I felt an overwhelming sense of relief, and although I desperately just wanted to stare at the girls' faces and listen to their voices, my body was exhausted—I'm sure partially from driving all day but also just with the knowledge that I was finally where I belonged. We went to bed early. Lying in my own bed next to my going-to-be-all-right husband was probably the greatest feeling ever.

We got up much sooner the next morning than I would have preferred. It was time for reality. I desperately wanted just to stay and bask in the feeling of being home, but there were things to do. First up: we had to get Blaine's driver's license renewed. He hated that he would be bald in his picture, but at least his beard was mostly back.

Eventually we finished at the DMV, and I went with him to his office to help unload his computer and all of the things he had taken to Texas so he could work from there. We walked in the door, and his coworkers jumped up to say hello and to help carry in his equipment. They all seemed so happy to see him, and I know Blaine was thrilled to be back. I, however, was feeling more and more anxious. I was so uncomfortable leaving him there! What if he got too tired? He was still sometimes a little unsteady on his feet. What if he fell? What if he got confused with so many people talking to him? (He was really past this issue at this point, but I still worried.) What if one of them was sick, and he caught their germs? For heaven's sake, what if one of them had COVID?

The owner of the company caught my eye and must have been able to tell how I was feeling. She put her arm around me and said, "It's okay. We'll take care of him." I was still pretty uncomfortable, but that did make me feel a little better. I kissed him goodbye and walked back to the car alone. My day was just getting started.

The next stop was to return the Mustard Seed to its rightful owner. Miraculously, Faith was going to arrive home the next day. After being gone for a year, somehow her first trip home was scheduled for the day after we would no longer need her car. Only God could have orchestrated that so perfectly! Even more amazing is that she was scheduled to return to the mission field the day before we needed to return to Houston for Blaine's surgery and had insisted we use it again. I couldn't get over the timing!

Unfortunately, my last stop of the day was to attend the funeral for a friend's husband. While I was thankful I was in town and could be there to support her, I felt very uncomfortable. I was there knowing my husband, who certainly could have died, was going to be fine, while her husband, who had been totally fine, had somehow died. This would not be the last time I would feel this way. Surviving is sometimes an awkward accomplishment.

The next morning, Kamryn and I made the six-hour drive to Ames, Iowa, to get Kaia and bring her home for Thanksgiving. I hadn't seen her since the middle of July and could not wait to wrap my arms around her and then bring her home for a few days so we could all be together!

By the time we made it back home the next evening, I should have been completely exhausted. Driving more than twenty-four hours in four days is not my idea of a good time, but it was so worth it, and I felt great! My family would all sleep in their own beds for the first time in months. I knew the week we had with Kaia would zip by too fast, but I was determined to enjoy every second. The next day, Blaine's father, stepmother, and sister came, and we celebrated Christmas. It was so fun to do it early, and watching Blaine's family see him looking so much better was priceless.

Soon it was the night before Thanksgiving. I had purchased a few things to prepare, but I was watching our money so carefully, and honestly, I was struggling to plan anything. It was as if my brain had handled all the problem-solving it was capable of and had somehow just checked out. We were sitting on the couch watching a movie when I got a text from a friend that said, "Go look on your porch."

I walked outside and discovered an entire Thanksgiving dinner cooked and ready to go! All I had to do was warm it up. She and her husband had left a note saying they loved us and didn't want us to worry about a thing on the holiday. It was such an awesome surprise! I carried it in, and everyone gathered around to see, ooohing and ahhhing over the delicious food. I walked out of the room to get something, and when I returned, Blaine was snacking on the turkey and raving about how great it tasted. I just stared at him, completely amazed. A few weeks ago, I had literally been crying and begging him to take a few sips of Ensure, and now he was chowing down on turkey after he had already eaten a full meal—and it tasted good! After all the months of everything tasting too salty, this was huge!

I woke up Thanksgiving morning feeling different than ever before. I've always been a pretty thankful person. I have kept a thankfulness list for years that literally has thousands of lines, but Thanksgiving felt different this year. I was completely overwhelmed with the blessings we had received. Sure, it had been an awful, awful year, but the way the Lord had taken care of even the tiniest details to make our situation as easy as possible and the unbelievable generosity of our family and friends, not just with monetary gifts, but the physical gifts we had received to make the situation more bearable, the acts of service, the phone calls, texts, and cards letting us know we weren't forgotten, filled me with a level of thankfulness I have never felt before. I sat at my table with all of my children and my husband, who was just a little bit more normal every day, and ate a dinner prepared by people who loved us. It was a happy Thanksgiving indeed.

Chapter 45

As I knew it would, our three weeks at home went by all too quickly, and soon we were on our way back to Houston. Somehow it felt even harder to leave this time than it had in June. Every day Blaine was scheduled for at least one appointment. He was to meet with the orthopedic surgeon, the plastic surgeon, and the anesthesia team, and he was to have blood work, an MRI of his arm, and the dreaded CT scan of his chest. This was the most worrisome because it would show if any sarcoma cells had formed in his lungs. We weren't expecting anything based on how effective the chemotherapy had been against Lumpy, but sarcomas are sneaky and unpredictable, so we were a little apprehensive. Blaine had been dreading undergoing another MRI, but when the time came, he was back to his normal, anxiety-free self and didn't have any problems.

The hospital never reported imaging results online, but I was excited for his labs to be posted. Blaine seemed so fine that I wasn't anticipating any issues, and I was looking forward to seeing good, healthy numbers. I didn't get them.

"Ummmmm . . . I think we may have a problem," I said as I finished reading through the list.

"Nope. No problems allowed. We are done with problems," Blaine replied.

"Both your platelets and your white count are still too low." My stomach began to churn as I realized what that would likely mean. Low platelets put him at increased risk of bleeding, and the low white count put him at increased risk of infection. I was afraid they would have to postpone the surgery, which would obviously mess up our Christmas plans, as well as potentially our deductible situation. I couldn't believe it! We were so close to being done. The thought that we might not finish on my timetable made me sick to my stomach.

Thankfully, we had an appointment with Dr. Knobloch, the orthopedic surgeon, later that day. She got right to the point: "Your chest looks perfectly clear!"

Whew! The biggest worry was taken care of!

"Your lab numbers aren't perfect, but I don't anticipate any problems."

Whew! Worry number two was over.

"The MRI shows the tumor has shrunk tremendously since your first one! This truly is amazing! Sarcomas typically do respond some to the chemo, but not nearly this dramatically."

Thank you, God!

"Unfortunately, your MRI shows the tumor is adhered to your cephalic vein. I'm going to have to cut that out when I take the tumor."

"How will that affect my function?"

"It probably won't. We'll need to watch it closely, though, because the cephalic vein is important for drainage of fluid in your arm. You could potentially have permanent swelling of your hand if we don't catch it quickly. Keep an eye on it."

We assured her we would. Somehow, I hadn't given any thought to the fact that he could have residual effects after the surgery besides the scar, but some swelling in his hand really seemed like a minor issue considering he could have lost his arm, not to mention his life.

"How soon after the surgery will he be able to drive?" I asked.

"Eight weeks."

This was not at all what Blaine was hoping to hear. He tried to bluff his way to a different response. "*A* week? That's not bad. I can do *a* week."

"No, no, no," she said. "*Eight* weeks. If you would need to make any sudden moves with your arm, you could rip the internal stitches, and since you'll be eleven hours away, I wouldn't be able to fix it. No driving for *eight* weeks. It must have time to heal correctly."

"Okay. I promise not to drive for *a* week."

"No, *EIGHT* weeks!" Dr. Knobloch, her nurse practitioner, and her student all said, laughing. "*EIGHT* weeks! *EIGHT* weeks! *EIGHT* weeks!"

"Okay, okay, okay," Blaine said with a grin. "I won't drive for *a* week!"

I rolled my eyes. "He'll be good. I promise." They all laughed. They thought he was hilarious.

The next day we met with the plastic surgeon for the first time. He explained the different ways he might need to close the incision after Dr. Knobloch had finished excising Lumpy. The best-case scenario was that he would just be able to stitch the incision closed, but if too much skin had to be removed, then it would be necessary to take a skin graft from Blaine's back to repair the spot. He did this type of closure on a regular basis and was not anticipating any issues, but it would definitely prolong the healing time.

We then met briefly with the anesthesia team. They examined Blaine to ensure there weren't any glaring issues that would complicate putting him under, and then we headed out for a celebratory dinner. Tomorrow at that time, Blaine would be cancer-free!

Chapter 46

We were up and on our way before the sun rose the next morning. Blaine seemed very calm, like it was just another day. I was so excited, I felt I might jump out of my skin. After eight traumatic months, Lumpy was finally going to be taken away! I love being outside before most people are awake, and our drive to the hospital was easy and peaceful. It's Houston, so of course there were cars on the road but considerably fewer than normal.

We found a parking spot easily, grabbed our things, and hurried to the door. Somehow, we were running just a little bit later than planned, but we were on the premises now and knew we'd be on the surgical floor in just a few more minutes. Blaine reached out to open the door. It was locked! What in the world? A guard walked by inside. She saw us looking panicked and came to help.

"Are you here for surgery?" she asked. We told her we were. "I'm sorry, but these doors don't open until 7. You'll have to go through the main entrance." The main entrance was kind of a trek from where we were. I was thankful Blaine was feeling better because we would have to move fast! We rushed around the building to the main entrance, passed the COVID guards, and finally made it to the elevator that would take us to the surgery floor. It was going to be close, but as long as there was no line to check in, we wouldn't be late.

The elevator door slid open. We stepped out and stared in complete shock. There were probably forty patients already there! We stood there for a moment with our mouths hanging open while the people in line smiled at us sympathetically, surely feeling thankful they had managed to arrive earlier. We took our place at the end of the line and slowly inched forward as the desk staff checked in more and more people and took them to the preoperative holding area.

Finally, it was Blaine's turn. He answered all the questions, and a tech led us back to his assigned bed. They handed him a gown to change into and gave him a big bag to hold all of his belongings. Blaine changed, put his things in the bag, and climbed into the bed to wait. Soon his nurse came to introduce herself.

"Mr. Parker? My name is Carly. I'll be taking care of you until they take you back for surgery. Can you tell me your medical record number and date of birth?"

Blaine rattled them both off. He had probably recited those numbers 10,000 times in the last six months.

"And what surgery are you having today?"

"I'm here for breast augmentation surgery."

I had just taken a sip of water and almost spit it out all over the floor.

Carly had actually started to write that on the chart but caught herself. "I'm sorry. What did you say?"

"Breast augmentation surgery. I need bigger boobs."

I burst out laughing.

"Okay, okay. I'm just here to get this one cut off." He pulled up his sleeve and gave her a good look at Lumpy.

Carly laughed. "That makes more sense. You had me going there for a minute! I'll be right back. I just need to grab the stuff for your IV." I heard her giggling as she walked away.

She was back a few minutes later and started the IV. Soon Dr. Knobloch came by to check on Blaine and to describe once more what she would be doing. Shortly after she left, the anesthesiologist came in to say hello and to see if Blaine had any questions. He didn't. We were just ready to get it over with.

Thankfully, we didn't have to wait long. Soon the transport team was there, and I kissed Blaine goodbye. It hadn't occurred to me until that very moment something might go wrong with the surgery, and I had a brief moment of panic as they wheeled him away. I prayed the first of my three million prayers of the day and felt better. Carly took me out to the waiting room. She showed me where I could lock up my things and introduced me to the volunteer who manned the waiting room desk. She also explained the monitors hanging in the corners. I could glance up at any time, find Blaine's medical record number, and know exactly what part of the procedure was happening.

I found a reasonably comfy chair and settled in for my long day of waiting. I texted a few people to let them know the surgery had started and made a Facebook post about what a crazy year it had been. I attached pictures of Kaia, Kaci, and Blaine on their gurneys awaiting their surgeries. It was hard to believe all that had happened to us in the last nine months.

Family and friends started texting about how they wished they could sit with me, and suddenly tears stung my eyes. I hadn't given any thought to the fact that if we were home, I wouldn't be sitting there by myself, but suddenly I felt so lonely! I looked around the waiting room and was reminded that every single person there was alone, thanks to the COVID restrictions. I was still sad, but realizing I wasn't alone in my loneliness somehow made it more tolerable.

Dr. Knobloch had told us she expected her portion of the surgery to take around five hours, and about five hours later she walked in and asked me to follow her into a little conference room. "Mrs. Parker! The surgery went very, very well! We took extensive margins and had pathology test them before I left. All of the margins were clear. We got all of the cancer! "

My knees almost buckled as relief swept over me. "Oh! That's incredible to hear. Thank you so, so much," I gushed as I hugged her.

"As expected, I did have to take the cephalic vein, but I don't anticipate him having any trouble."

"That's okay. We'll watch it. I'm not worried."

"The tumor looked even better than I was hoping. It is extremely rare for a sarcoma to respond as well as his did to treatment. It's a miracle really."

"We have a big God," I replied, beaming and overwhelmed with the truth of this.

She smiled and said, "Yes, we do."

Then she started laughing, "We heard he told the nurse he was here for breast augmentation surgery! We were all chuckling about that all through the operation! Your husband is so funny!"

I agreed. He's a hoot. I knew he would love hearing he made everyone laugh.

We had cleared the beach trip with her earlier. She remembered this and told me to have a great time. I gushed my thanks to her again and wished her a wonderful Christmas. We had a conference call scheduled for the first week of January, when the official pathology report of Lumpy would be in, so I knew I would talk to her again soon. She left to prepare for her next surgery, and I went back to my chair. I knew the plastic surgeon was closing him now, but I did not know how involved that would be or how long it would take.

About an hour later, I heard my name being called and looked up to see the plastic surgeon waiting for me. I followed him into the little conference room. "Good news!" he said. "We were able to close Blaine up without doing a skin graft. The incision covers most of his upper arm, but it should heal without any problems. If everything goes as I expect, he should be able to leave the hospital tomorrow. We'll take the stitches and the drain out in two weeks, and you can go home!"

I thanked him and walked back to my chair. It was over! Those words kept replaying in my mind. *It was over!* I was a little afraid I was just dreaming. My body immediately wanted a nap, and I worried I might fall asleep right in the waiting room, but frankly, I didn't even care. It was over. My husband was going to be fine, and we were going back to our lives.

I knew I wouldn't see him until he was out of recovery and in his room for the night, so I waited patiently. I waited and waited and waited. Finally, I gave in and asked the volunteer if she could find out what was going on. She came back a few minutes later and said they were having trouble finding a room for him because the hospital was so full. This was a problem I certainly hadn't anticipated! It didn't really matter. I knew they would figure it out eventually. Nothing mattered. My husband was going to be fine! I was pretty sure nothing would bother me ever again.

I sat in the waiting room for a few more hours, and then finally someone came to get me. "We're sorry it's taking so long," she said. "It's against the rules for you to be in the recovery room, but we're making an exception. We'll get him sent to a room as soon as possible, but in the meantime, you should be together."

I thanked her and followed her into the recovery area. I could hear a woman screaming. That was a little unnerving, but thankfully I turned the corner to see Blaine's smiling face! He looked a little sleepy but otherwise fine. All the anesthesia had worn off, and he was completely coherent, but thankfully, they had given him enough medication to ensure he was pain-free. He had a huge bandage, and his arm was in a sling. I was curious to know what the incision looked like but at the same time not really wanting to see it.

The woman kept screaming.

The patient across from Blaine hadn't been out of surgery as long. The nurse walked up to check something, and he said, "Hi, I'm John. What's going on?"

"You just had surgery," the nurse explained to him. "We're going to send you up to your room in a little bit."

"Oh! Really? Okay." He seemed so surprised.

The woman kept screaming.

A few minutes later, the nurse walked by again. The man said, "Hi, I'm John. What's going on?" The nurse told him he had just had surgery. "Oh! Really? Okay."

The woman kept screaming.

This scenario replayed over and over. I was so impressed with the nurse. Not once did he sound at all irritated. He just answered the question like it was the first time every time.

The woman kept screaming.

I finally asked the nurse if she was okay. "Oh, yes. She's totally fine. Sometimes people just do that when they are first waking up."

I was beginning to understand why they don't allow caregivers in the recovery room.

A room finally opened up, and they took Blaine upstairs. I followed along. It was well after visiting hours had ended, but I stayed and helped him eat some dinner. It was pretty difficult for him not to be able to use his arm at all, but we knew he would adjust quickly. Finally, there was nothing left for me to do, so I kissed him goodnight and drove back to the Cottage. I fell into bed and slept better than I probably have in my entire life. Everything was finally right. *It was over.*

Chapter 47

Reasonably early the next morning, Blaine called and said he was going to be discharged in a few hours. Dr. Knobloch had originally predicted he would need to stay in the hospital for five days after the surgery, so being able to have him back home that day was amazing! I fiddled around the Cottage until it was time to go to the hospital. I couldn't wait to see him!

I walked into his room, and a gigantic grin took over my face when I saw him up and moving. His arm was still heavily bandaged and resting in a black sling, and there was a drain tube coming out of the skin near his elbow, but other than that he seemed completely fine. He was talking and happy and ready to go. An occupational therapist came and showed us the best way to get his shirt on and off without moving his arm too much, and the nurse had us watch a video demonstrating how to empty his drain. The fluid had to be removed every morning and every evening, and I needed to record how much came out and what his temperature was. The video was well done, and I felt completely prepared. They sent him home with three different types of pain medicine, anti-inflammatory medication, and an antibiotic. Six months ago, I would have felt intimidated by the thought of keeping track of all those, but compared to what he had been taking while he was on the chemo, this medicine regimen seemed like nothing.

We went back to the Cottage and I got him settled in. He was already learning to do things with one hand. We ate dinner and watched some TV, and then it was time to check his temperature and empty his drain. He stood by the kitchen sink while I washed my hands and grabbed an alcohol wipe. I followed the directions we had been shown on the video, dragging the blood and pus down the tube into the reservoir. I was focusing on getting it all out of the tube when all of a sudden, Blaine lurched forward. I paused and looked up. He was white as a ghost! "Are you okay?"

"I don't . . . feel . . . so good." He started to fall forward.

I caught him and slowly helped him over to a kitchen chair. We sat there for a long time, waiting for his lightheadedness to pass. Eventually, he felt better, and I finished stripping the drain. I recorded the amount of fluid and then poured it down the toilet. I helped him get into bed and lay down beside him.

It was definitely not over.

I hadn't been prepared for how weak he would be or how scary it would be to care for him. I should have been. I had cared for Kaia and Kaci after their surgeries, and I knew Blaine obviously was in much poorer health than they were, but it caught me completely by surprise. I had convinced myself it was all over and life would be easy now that Lumpy was gone. I sighed and resigned myself to the fact we weren't quite there yet as I set multiple alarms for his various nighttime meds. "One day closer . . . one day closer," I said over and over to myself as I dozed off to sleep.

The next morning it was time to change his dressing. I was terrified of hurting him, but it had to be done. The first step was to take off his shirt. It was a little complicated, but we figured it out, and soon we could change his shirt without even really thinking about it.

Once Blaine's shirt was off, I finally got a good look at his arm. A translucent adhesive bandage covered the skin from his elbow almost to his shoulder. Under that was a long, thick piece of bloody gauze. I tried to be cool and reassuring as I cautiously began peeling off the bandage and the gauze, but an involuntary gasp escaped when I saw the incision. It looked so much worse than I was expecting! It reminded me of a long, curvy, puckered-up caterpillar, the stitches resembling randomly placed black legs poking out. It got flatter further down near the elbow, but the whole thing looked shockingly bad. I slowly released my breath and reminded myself that it didn't matter. Lumpy was gone. Nothing else was important.

I emptied the drain and recorded all the details. I carefully wiped away the dried blood around the incision site with an alcohol wipe, and then Blaine got into the shower. We had learned from the experience the night before and put a chair in the shower. I'm not sure he needed it, but I felt much better knowing it was there just in case.

When he was finished, I helped him dry off, and then, as instructed, put Neosporin around the wound to help it heal and then covered it with a new bandage. He got dressed and lay down for a nap. All we had done that morning was take care of his basic needs, but it was exhausting for both of us.

Chapter 48

When we arrived back at the Cottage after our brief trip home for Thanksgiving, we discovered Lydia had decorated it for Christmas! There was even a full-size Christmas tree with lights and ornaments. We had wrapped all the presents before Blaine's surgery, and they were waiting under the tree. Now all we needed were our girls! The day finally arrived for Kaci and Kamryn's flight. After picking them up from the airport, we took the long way back to show them the best Christmas lights. Houston may have grueling traffic and unbearably muggy weather, but its residents sure know how to decorate!

Kaia's practice schedule kept her in Iowa a bit longer, but two days later, we loaded up the Mustard Seed and headed for the airport to complete our family. We had all been together the week of Thanksgiving, but I was still so excited! Having all five of us together will always be my favorite thing, and this time it felt extra special.

We squeezed Kaia and her luggage into the car and headed for the beach! Kaia has always been a warm-weather lover. The weather in southern Texas is very different from that of central Iowa, and it was so fun to watch her bloom. We chatted all the way down, and before we knew it, we were crossing the bridge that connects Galveston Island to the mainland. The rest of us had been there a few months earlier, but Kaia hadn't seen the ocean in years. I was so thankful we could be together for Christmas. That we were together at the *beach* for Christmas made it even better!

As I pulled into the address Lydia had given me, my mouth fell open. I was silent, but the girls were whooping with excitement. We were at a luxury resort! There were huge ocean-facing windows everywhere we looked and stunning Christmas decorations. There were restaurants and a spa and a gorgeous pool and hot tub where we could soak while we watched the waves. We went up to the top floor where Lydia's place was located and unlocked the door to discover glass walls in every room with a breathtaking ocean view. She had even snuck down at some point and put up a little Christmas tree for us to enjoy while we were there. The whole thing was over-the-top gorgeous, and I was stunned that it was ours for the next four days.

Blaine, being the beach-hater he is, settled himself on the couch to watch a movie, but the rest of us rushed down to get our toes in the water. We spent as much of the next four days as possible directly on the beach, on our balcony overlooking the beach, or in the hot tub staring at the beach. We knew it would likely be a long time before we saw the ocean again, and we didn't want to waste a minute. It had been an incredibly stressful year for all of us, but the sound of waves breaking against the sand might be the best therapy there is.

Christmas morning, Kamryn and I got up early and were on the beach in time to watch the sunrise. She loves taking photographs, and I love watching her take photographs. It was a beautiful time I'll never forget. Eventually, we went back inside for our traditional Christmas breakfast and to unwrap a few presents. I snapped a photo of the girls in front of the window overlooking the ocean, with stockings Lydia had made for them and the little tree. It was definitely not our normal Christmas photo, but it was so much more meaningful. God had provided and blessed us in ways we never could have imagined, and that photo will be displayed in our home every Christmas to ensure we don't forget.

All too soon, it was time to leave. We took the girls to the airport and watched them walk away from us again. I was sad but knew we would see them soon. This whole ordeal was almost over, and we would be back to our real life.

We all settled back into our routines. Blaine and I picked our work back up at the little table in the Cottage; Kaia resumed her practice schedule, and Kaci and Kamryn went back home to wait for Blaine and me to arrive. They were in between school semesters, so they didn't have much to do.

As it often happens when people have extra time on their hands, particularly when they're living through stressful times, little irritations become big annoyances. Kaci and Kamryn love each other, but sibling bickering had become common. It's hard to mediate from six hundred miles away, and I had learned to just stay out of it whenever I could. One day I was helping Lydia with an errand when I realized I had missed a call from Kaci. As I was telling Lydia I needed to return her call, Kamryn called. I sighed. When they both called, it meant they were fighting, and each wanted me to take her side and tell the other one to get it together. I decided to ignore them both. It was exhausting, and I just didn't have it in me to deal with it that day.

Soon Kaci called again. Then Kamryn. Then Kaci. "Oh boy," I thought, "this must be a doozy." I considered just turning off my phone, but Blaine was at the Cottage by himself, and I wanted to know he could get a hold of me if he needed something. Soon they resorted to texting, and my phone started dinging over and over. *Mom! Mom! Mom!* I ignored it.

Finally, I gave up and glanced down to read Kaci's text. It said, "LUMPY IS HERE! HELP!"

What in the world? I called her. She picked up on the first ring. "MOM! They sent Lumpy here. It came in a box and said it's supposed to be frozen immediately. *Why* is it here? Am I really supposed to just keep it in the *freezer*????"

Of all the issues I thought they might be having, I certainly was not expecting this! For a moment I was too stunned to even reply, but slowly realized there was no way they would send a cancerous tumor to someone's home! "It can't be Lumpy. Tell me what the box says."

"Specimen enclosed. Freeze immediately."

It took me a few minutes, but I finally figured it out. Blaine had agreed to participate in a study to help researchers learn about sarcomas. They mentioned they would be sending a box for him to mail back a stool sample. There must have been a miscommunication about where to send it. I burst out laughing. I could hear Kamryn in the background. They were both freaking out! I knew I shouldn't laugh, but there was no way to hold it in. I wished I had been there so I could actually see their faces when they thought they were holding Lumpy!

I explained what it was. Kaci felt better but was still pretty grossed out. They made room in the freezer for the box and tried not to think about it. I, however, told the story over and over. They'll never live it down!

Blaine seemed to have a little more energy and a little less pain every day. As unbelievable as it seemed, the day finally arrived for the stitches and drain to be removed, and then we could actually head home for good. We packed everything in the car and tearfully said goodbye to Lydia. In addition to meeting our physical needs, she had provided the emotional and spiritual support we so desperately needed. She had become our friend, and we would miss her so much.

We sat down in the plastic surgeon's exam room, and his assistant pulled out the drain and all the stitches, and just like that, we were done! I was afraid I might be dreaming, but it was real! My whole body felt lighter. My steps actually felt bouncy, and I could not keep from grinning like I had just won the lottery. Truthfully, I *had* won the lottery, and I knew it.

I texted the girls and posted to the Facebook group that we were heading home, and we jumped in the Mustard Seed. The doctors insisted we take a break every couple of hours to let Blaine walk around and that we stop halfway and spend the night so he would not get a blood clot. He was frustrated with this, as he just wanted to be home, but it would have been a long, uncomfortable trip if we had tried to do it all in one day, and I was glad the doctors had made us break it up.

Pulling into our garage the next day was without a doubt one of the greatest moments of my life. It was over. We were home!

Chapter 49

A week later we were scheduled to have a conference call with Dr. Knobloch and her assistant to go over Lumpy's pathology report. Blaine had missed so much work over the last six months that we decided I would drive to his office, and we would just talk with them in the car. I felt a weird combination of excited anticipation and terror. Blaine climbed in the car, and we made nervous chitchat while we waited for the phone to ring. Thankfully it didn't take long.

"Hello, Mr. and Mrs. Parker! I have amazing news for you *again*!" I let out the breath I had been unknowingly holding since the phone rang. I was so thankful she never waited to let us know if her news was good or bad. "The pathology report is back for Blaine's tumor. It confirmed it was an extremely aggressive cancer, *but* it was 99 percent dead when they removed it and there were *no signs* of cancer around it. There is less than a 10 percent chance of recurrence. I have already spoken with Dr. Baldyga, and she will not be recommending that you do any more chemotherapy."

My mind was reeling. Ninety-nine percent dead? Less than 10 percent chance of recurrence? No more chemotherapy? Dr. Knobloch reminded us again how those results were very rare for sarcomas, particularly ones this aggressive. There was not a doubt in my mind that God had personally annihilated Lumpy. He had used the people at MDA to do it, but ultimately, He was the one responsible, and there was no way I could ever thank Him enough.

"How is your arm feeling?" she asked Blaine.

"Good! It's a little bit stiff and sore, but basically it's fine."

"I'm so glad! Be sure to move it around a lot. We can give you a referral for physical therapy if you would like. Just let us know. You're not driving, are you?"

"Of course I am. You said I only had to wait *a* week."

I heard them both gasp. "Mr. Parker!"

"He's not driving!" I interjected. "Don't worry. He's being good."

I could hear them laughing. I wondered if all their patients were this difficult.

We planned out our next visit with them. Even though there was a low likelihood of recurrence, because it was such an aggressive tumor, if it did come back, it could spread quickly, so they would need to take images of his arm and chest every three months for the next two years and every six months for at least three more years after that. That was a lot of very expensive/inconvenient trips to Texas, but it seemed like a small price to pay to ensure we could catch it before it spread. Dr. Knobloch and Dr. Baldyga would alternate their visits. In three months, Blaine would see Dr. Baldyga and then three months after that, Dr. Knobloch.

They reminded Blaine again that he was not allowed to drive for five more weeks, we said goodbye, and then just like that, it was truly over. Well, it was over for three months, but we were now looking at three whole months of normal life. I texted the girls to tell them the amazing results of the pathology report and then posted to the Facebook group. I felt like I could really breathe for the first time in the last eight months, and I drove straight home and took a long nap.

Chapter 50

Just a few days earlier we had turned the calendar and started a brand-new year. I truly felt like a new person. I had learned so much in the last eight months, and I knew I would never be the same. I wanted to somehow document all I had learned, so I posted these comments on Facebook for everyone to read.

1. Day to day "normal" stressors don't matter. I used to get so stressed about completely unimportant stuff. Struggling every day to keep your favorite person alive while being six hundred-plus miles from all your other favorite people makes worrying about whether or not the kitchen is clean or someone's algebra homework is done seem completely idiotic. I'm really hoping I can keep this perspective (well, maybe not about the homework, but you get my point).

2. I very clearly saw God use something that seemed really awful for our good. We had been praying so hard the doctor would know exactly how much chemo Blaine needed, but there was no way she was going to deviate from the basic treatment plan. It took Blaine's reacting really badly to make her stop it. While we had been praying so hard Blaine wouldn't suffer side effects, God was busy using those side effects to make sure he got the correct amount of chemo.

3. God really will meet our needs when we have no way of meeting them ourselves. Of course, I always said I believed that, but now I know for sure it's true. The way our financial needs were met shocked us, and frankly the physical strength He gave me to get through the multiple nights in a row when I needed to be able to respond quickly to Blaine's needs, physically and intellectually, with little to no sleep was miraculous as well.

I believed all of that with all my heart. It was true. I knew it was true, but somehow, all of that confidence just slowly slid away. Blaine seemed to adjust easily back to our real life. He continued to have neuropathy in his toes, and eventually his toenails all just completely flaked off, and for a few months he did sometimes continue to slur his words, which he found embarrassing. Other than that, he just jumped right back into life as if nothing had ever happened.

I, however, did not. For the first six weeks we were home, I caught every single germ that came anywhere near me and was sick over and over. Then, as the days moved forward, I began to feel more and more detached. I felt out of place all the time, like I no longer belonged in my own life. Every morning I expected to wake up and discover we were still in Texas, still in the thick of his treatment and all the unknowns. Kaci and Kamryn adjusted shockingly well to having to share the house and follow our rules and schedule again, but I would be lying if I said there weren't a few bumps, and these were painful reminders of the time I had lost with them, time I would never get back.

I even felt awkward with my friends. Blaine and I went to a party shortly after returning home. I could hear him downstairs with all the men, laughing and having a great time. I was upstairs with the women, acting fine, but inside I was so uncomfortable! I felt so out of place, as if I were really no longer part of the group.

To make matters worse, the medical bills started flooding in. While we had met our deductible for the previous year, Blaine had to have repeat scans; Kaci needed more physical therapy, and Kamryn developed mysterious abdominal pain that required expensive tests and then surgery. I had stressed so much about finishing all of Blaine's treatments in the last calendar year, but the reality was we started right over once January hit. Blaine was always going to require expensive testing. Even if the cancer never came back, the costs involved in making sure he was okay were going to eat us alive every single year.

While we were in Texas, I had started experiencing the odd phenomenon of somehow personally feeling other people's pain, and this continued after we returned home. If anything unpleasant happened to anyone around me, I felt as if it were happening to me. Between my own pressures and absorbing everyone else's, I felt as if I were being physically hit over and over every single day, week after week, month after month. I kept thinking surely I would adjust, but every day, it seemed like there was a new problem and things that should have just been a little inconvenience felt like an insurmountable situation that was going to ruin my life.

I was so sad all the time, and it completely baffled me. I finally had exactly what I had been praying so desperately for. It didn't make any sense, but I woke up in the morning sad, I dragged myself through every day feeling sad, and I lay awake at night unable to sleep because I was so sad. This was complicated by guilt. What right did I have to feel sad? What was wrong with me? I hadn't lost my husband. We had stared death in the eye and come out relatively unscathed. I didn't have anything to grieve. I have always considered myself to be a mentally tough person. I had never felt anything like this before. Why couldn't I get it together?

Slowly, it hit me. I had suffered loss. I had lost the illusion that we were young and healthy and serious disease was something we didn't have to worry about. I had lost the illusion that I was essential for my children's wellbeing. I had lost the illusion that we would retire comfortably one day with money to do things we wanted. I had lost the illusion that I had any control over my life at all.

Realizing it wasn't ridiculous for me to grieve helped me to feel a little better. About this time, I also remembered my friend Traci's comment about adrenal fatigue. I did some research and discovered I had all the symptoms, and the most common cause: I had been too stressed for too long. I talked to my doctor, who advised that I make more of an effort to take care of myself physically, eating healthy food and getting enough sleep and exercise. I also started taking a supplement that supported my adrenal glands. It took a long time, way longer than I would have imagined, but eventually, I did get myself back.

You've come to the part of the story where I'm supposed to tell you all I've learned and how wonderful it all is. It is wonderful.

It's also hard.

There are always going to be fears about the cancer returning or someone getting hurt. There are always going to be money problems.

There is also going to be joy and laughter and wonderful surprises that take our breath away.

I'm going to focus on savoring the perfect moments, and I'm going to push through the hard stuff; I'm going to be intentional about loving my people and other people's people, and I'm going to trust that God, who knows way more than I do, loves me and has my back, even if I may not always understand.

How to Support Someone Going Through a Crisis

I surveyed individuals dealing with various crises about ways people could help them. Below are the most common responses:

1. Overwhelmingly, people told me they needed their friends and family to continue talking to them. They need their friends and family to stick with them, to continue telling them about their lives and asking them about theirs. Continue to invite them to things, even if you know they probably won't be able to go. It's always nice to know you're wanted. Be a friend, even if you feel uncomfortable. Trust me, your friend facing the crisis is uncomfortable too. Don't make it worse by abandoning them.

2. Do not just ask what you can do to help. I'm sure anything you can think of will be helpful. Don't make the person going through the crisis come up with the idea or have to verbalize it. Just do something.

3. Give money. Checks, cash, and gift cards are all great. Don't ask if they need it. Trust me, they do. If you have the means, paying off a bill, even if it's not a large one, helps tremendously both

financially and mentally.

4. Provide meals that are either already prepared or easy-to-warm-up freezer meals. While someone is actively undergoing chemotherapy, lighter, more bland meals might be best for them. The caregiver, on the other hand, deserves something yummy!

5. Bring groceries. (It is okay to call and ask what they need.)

6. Clean their house.

7. Do their laundry.

8. Mow their grass/take care of their yard.

9. Mail them cards. Just knowing someone is thinking of you means so much.

10. Send texts reminding them you care.

11. Listen closely to the side effects the patient is experiencing and think about products that might make them more comfortable (for example, a Snuggie if they are struggling with feeling cold).

12. Educate yourself so you know what they are experiencing. Explaining things over and over is exhausting.

13. Pray! Pray for healing. Pray for comfort. Pray for peace. Pray for provision. Let them know you are praying. There is huge comfort in this.

14. After you have proven you are willing to help with the basics, let it be known that you are there for other random things the family might need (and then follow through if they ask).

Endnotes

1. I should note here that since this whole experience, I have done way too much research into soft tissue sarcomas on the extremities. Every single story I have read or heard started out with a doctor misdiagnosing it. Every single one. I have struggled with anger toward this doctor, but I don't think it's his fault. There simply must be more education.

2. When the bill finally arrived for the ultrasound, it was $80. That was a huge lesson for us, and we vowed to never pay upfront for any medical procedures again.

3. I look back on this moment now and laugh. Over the next few months, we would both learn so much humility. So many people helped us, and while we never got to the point where we were comfortable with that, we didn't have a choice but to accept it, and we were so, so very thankful.

4. The decision of who to tell and who not to tell was a big deal for us. We had several family members and close friends who were facing large issues themselves, and we did not want to add to their burdens. There were also people we knew would be extremely concerned, and it seemed unfair to make them worry before we knew exactly what Blaine was facing.

5. I have changed the name of this very well-respected hospital so it is not judged unfairly. It is an excellent hospital with brilliant physicians, and I would not hesitate to use it for other circumstances.

6. Just because we were unaware of other physicians reviewing Blaine's case does not mean that it didn't happen. I am almost certain now that it did.

7. The Bible says, "God can do anything, you know—far more than you could ever imagine or guess or request in your wildest dreams!" (Ephesians 3:20 MSG). I know this, of course, but sometimes it still surprises me.

8. In the end, different moms stepped in and provided driving lessons for Kamryn. We were home in time to give her lots of practice time, and now she's a great driver. I am so incredibly thankful for the "village" that took over when we needed them the most!

9. I've known people who were really sick and received transfusions of either whole blood or platelets, and they all felt like a totally new person the next day. I was always excited when Blaine got one because I expected him to have that sort of reaction too, but he never did. Honestly, we usually couldn't tell much of a difference at all.

10. Getting out of Blaine's room for a bit did so much for my emotional state that I did my best to get out for a little bit every day afterward. MD Anderson has a skywalk connecting the main building with another one. It has large windows that give one the sensation of being outside and is long enough to provide a little exercise. Walking on this skywalk is one of the best choices I made during this awful time.

11. The two men who worked the valet parking system for the radiation department were amazing. We interacted with them twice every weekday for five weeks, and every single time they were cheerful and encouraging and made us feel really good about being there. Many times, they would be overrun with cars and patients who all somehow arrived at the same time, but never once were they unpleasant, and they never ever made us feel rushed. Doctors and nurses tend to get all the credit, and obviously they are critically important, but the role the support staff make in the overall patient experience should be acknowledged more. These guys brightened our day every single time we saw them, and I am so thankful they are there!

Without a doubt, friends, family, and strangers we met along the way helped make this experience easier, but Jesus is the one who carried me. If you'd like to know more about Him, please visit ChristiParkerBooks.com

I hope you enjoyed our story! You can help reach even more people by leaving a quick review on Amazon. Thank you!

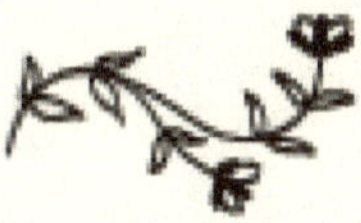

I would love to keep in touch! Visit ChristiParkerBooks.com where you can send me an email and sign up for my monthly newsletter to receive updates on new books and MORE!